MW00414458

Get continued support through Facebook.com/FlablesslyFit
and Twitter: @FlablesslyFit

Medifast &Me &You Unauthorized Evaluation

TED SALOIS

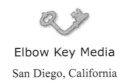

Elbow Key Media

San Diego, California

ISBN: 978-0-9915971-4-7

Elbow Key Media
8030 La Mesa Blvd. # 256, La Mesa, CA 91942
www.elbowkeymedia.com

Dedication

To my awesome wife, Yuko, who put up with my obscene level of bloated obesity for too long and showed great restraint and class by never calling me exactly what I was. Her great attention, care and cooking also were instrumental in my dieting success.

To my wonderful offspring (Rosanna, Momo and Jake) who seemed to care little about my appearance but provided unwavering support for my pursuit of a healthier body. My great hope is that my journey has taught them that we should eat to sustain life rather than achieve a desired level of comfort. The latter should be obtained through companionship of family and friends and by engaging in challenging mental and physical endeavors.

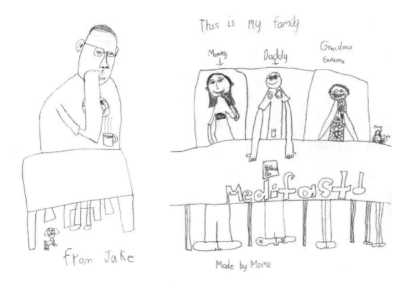

Warning:

Be sure to get clearance from your medical doctor
before beginning any diet program.

Disclaimers

This manuscript chronicles the author's participation in the prepackaged-food diet program known as Medifast, which is a trademark of Jason Enterprises, Inc.

Throughout the entire process of writing, publishing and distributing this book, THE AUTHOR HAD NO ASSOCIATION WITH THE DIET PLAN COMPANY or anyone connected to it other than his routine participation in its weight-loss program. He was merely a paying customer, exactly the same as anyone else who engages that organization seeking help to trim unwanted body fat. The diet company provided no sponsorship of the book project and had no knowledge of it during the duration of the author's participation.

Also, to clarify for anyone paying very close attention to the numbers recorded in the pages ahead: the author's initial weigh-in at the program office registered at 210 pounds. His scale at home showed him at 207. Throughout the program, this difference in readings remained consistent. The reason for the misalignment was not a matter of scale inaccuracy, however; it was because of the times of day when the author stepped onto the two mechanisms. His bathroom weight-check occurred regularly at about 6:30 a.m. His program office weigh-in took place a few hours later in the day. Such time variation always will produce slightly different numbers.

Lastly, the author's total weight loss actually was about 80 pounds. A visit to his doctor for non-weight-related items several months before he began the diet program registered at 219 pounds. When he completed the program, he was roughly 139 pounds. As noted above, the author was officially weighed by his program nutritionist at 210. He later tipped their scales at 142 when he transitioned off of the controlled program. Since this book focuses on the program diet traits and results, those latter numbers are considered to be the official count for the sake of this project.

Contents

Acknowledgments

Tristan Hayman, a successful veteran of the same diet plan, gave me insight into what to expect. In fact, it was his initial conversation with me that confirmed this was the program I would engage. It offered all the things I was looking for in a diet: plenty of meals that taste good, and a counselor who would be checking me frequently. Tristan didn't stop there, however. He continued to be a constant supporter with information and encouragement.

Tina Jenkins, a colleague whose keen eye for detail and enthusiasm for precision kept the words, sentences, paragraphs and pages herein at the proper place and appearing correctly. This project would have been seriously lacking had her professional influence not been leveled upon it.

Rick Rogers, former coworker and long-time friend, has been a steadfast source of helpful and interesting nutrition and exercise information. He remains eager to engage and continually encourages my participation in a variety of fun and fitness-maintaining sporting activities. I am looking forward to many more years of the same.

Steve Taylor, an old friend who always has been committed to eating right and exercising to stay in great shape, is a role model for such endeavors. Steve's unwavering pursuit of top conditioning has been an inspiration and aided in my decision to get serious about affecting the appropriate changes to my life.

Katharine Dizaye, a registered dietetic technician, was my counselor. I am very appreciative of her professionalism and extensive knowledge, which she freely shared with me. Katharine and all the other counselors at the diet program office in El Cajon, Calif., were extremely gracious and supportive throughout my weight-loss journey. I also saw them exhibit the same great customer service traits in dealing with a parade of other folks seeking help to slim their bodies. I tip my hat to the entire crew.

Dr. Erick Huang of Scripps Rancho San Diego Clinic in La Mesa, Calif., showed great diligence (as always) to explain things in great detail so that I had all the tools to make important decisions regarding actions to achieve and support my good health.

Introduction:
How to benefit from this book

The true value of following the weight-loss journey chronicled in the pages ahead lies beyond the diet company that made the foods the author consumed while losing 68 pounds in less than 6 months.

The reader will prosper most significantly by witnessing the numerous obstacles, mental and physical, the author faced and how he conquered them to achieve a weight and body shape he had not enjoyed since he was in high school.

Anyone embarking on a path to thin is certain to encounter similar difficulties. Seeing them tackled by the author will help the reader identify the method to advance past those rough points.

Knowledge gained from seeing these many small battles won is the essential tool the reader can use to accomplish a larger victory of substantial weight loss.

Weight loss similar or greater than that achieved by the author can be accomplished through almost any diet program.

The true hero in weight loss is the dieter, the one who gains the needed information and pursues the goal with hard-charging dedication.

Your emersion into this book is evidence of your determination. Go forth, shed all your unwanted pounds and enjoy extraordinary success.

How best to proceed

The author recommends the reader devour the entire text before beginning a diet program. The text was written in a style that should whisk the reader through to the end in nothing flat.

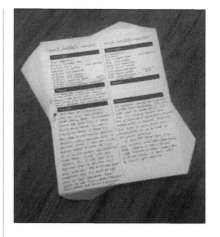

The author further suggests the dieter then follow his entries, day-for-day from the beginning, for a real-time comparison of events, actions, emotions, difficulties and achievements while recording all foods, exercises and comments in the dieter's own journal.

Forms are available for downloading from the author's website, **FlablesslyFit.com**. Keeping track of meals and fitness routines will assist the dieter in developing new, long-term habits to ensure proper weight is maintained for many years to come.

The author has kept his ideal weight since completing his diet program and attributes much of that success to the continued recording and tracking of his daily meals and activities. The author's website also offers articles on nutrition and exercise for program finishers who wish to continue learning and increasing their level of fitness beyond just accomplishing a particular, predetermined body weight.

The informative articles at **FlablesslyFit.com** invite comments and questions from readers. They also allow sharing of readers' success stories.

Best of luck in your journey. You won't need it, though. Knowledge, attitude and perserverence will get you thin!

Bon voyage.

How this book came to be

When I began the program, the good people at the diet company's local weight control center recommended that I participate with a buddy, a partner to encourage me if I showed signs of losing my enthusiasm. Since I had no friend who could serve in that capacity, I decided this writing project would act as my companion. I felt that committing to a book that required daily entries would help me with my commitment to the meals and exercise activities. I was right. It worked.

Even if you are able to convince someone to participate with you in your diet program, you should find great benefit in following me through this book, seeing what my experiences were a day or more ahead of your own. Also, I've made forms available you can fill in with your own comments about your experiences and reap the same reward that I did—all the while creating a permanent record of your incredible weight-loss adventure.

INSPIRATION

Sharing photos from the past was a popular, weekly ritual on social media. You may have heard of it: Throw Back Thursday or TBT. My participation in this game ran me across an old

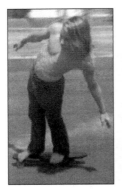 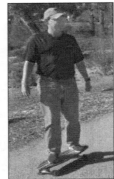 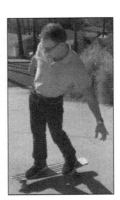

The young me   The round me   The new me

picture of me taken when I was a teenager. I looked at myself gliding along on a skateboard. What intrigued me was my super lean physique. I asked myself, "Why can't I be like that today?" I could think of no reasonable answer.

I had heard all the excuses about how there is no escaping weight gain as we age. Anyone who accepts such reasoning is just rationalizing a lack of desire to commit.

The evidence is out there. Plenty of examples can be found. People whose youth has slipped away are still able to achieve great fitness. And these are not the people whose metabolism just speedily burns off their calories.

People who pay careful attention to what they eat and stay active can maintain a slim body without difficulty. I know. I have become one of them.

I hope you join this group of extremely happy people.

Things to know before you begin

Miss no meals:

Logic says that eating less means fewer calories and faster weight loss. This is untrue, however. A proper diet program schedules the right number of calories to create a precise deficit.

If it is altered, the body will adjust and slow your overall calorie burn and weight loss.

It is vital to stick to the plan for the speediest possible success. Resist the temptation to reduce the prescribed number of meals.

Mental preparation is imperative:

Monitoring your weight is an essential element of any diet program. Once you are well into the program, however, you realize the scale plays tricks on you. Its readings will dance up and down and cause anguish.

I was warned about this activity. I was still unprepared for its true effect.

If you think it may help, declare to yourself—out loud in a stern voice—that you will prohibit these little fluctuations from dampening your enthusiasm.

Force yourself to concentrate on the overall trend, which will be downward, if you adhere to the requirements of the program.

If you find the saw-tooth pattern of weight readings still a serious bother to your psychological tranquility, another remedy is to jump onto the scale only at weekly intervals. This will always show a reduction in weight and ease your mind, as long as your mind allows you to get through the week on faith.

A couple of good results on a weekly basis should make that an easy acceptance.

Water at room temperature:

In the early stages of my program, I filled my 24-ounce bottle with ice before topping it off with water.

I was sure I needed it chilled. I felt I would be unable to enjoy the drink otherwise.

Then one day, I forgot my bottle at home. I had to drink store-bought water I had previously stashed at my office. I drank it straight... at room temperature.

I found the water went down much easier and faster since it was no shock to my throat. I realized ice was unnecessary. Its absence allowed me to consume the needed quantities—a full day's requirement—in less time and with no worry I would end the day short of my water goal.

Try your water without ice and see if you have a similarly beneficial experience.

Food selections:

It is worth pointing out a couple of important characteristics of the numerous packaged food items available to dieters in a variety of weight-loss programs.

Whether it is a mental or physical fact, you will want your selected meal choices to be filling.

I have found the packaged wild rice and chicken soup to be a favorite in this regard.

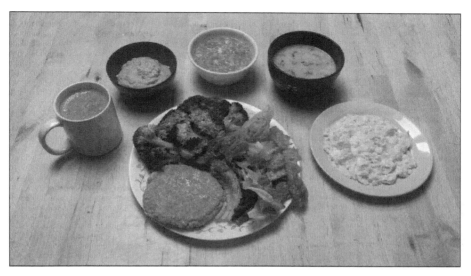

A typical day's food for me on my diet plan consisted of cappuccino, instant oatmeal, Maryland style crab-flavored soup, wild rice & chicken soup, scrambled eggs, and a normal, home-cooked dinner with lettuce, broccoli, zucchini, spinach and beef, chicken, fish or pork.

It is a little bland on its own, but a bit of spice solves that issue.

Also, the oatmeal choices are substantive and tasty, but I had to get past a prejudice for the texture.

I found I liked it.

Even if I hadn't, I probably would have worked this choice into my daily schedule because it has health benefits beyond its low-calorie status.

See the appendix for more information on the plan's packaged foods.

1

So it begins, turning desires into reality

The voice on the phone was friendly, maybe even cheerful. "Good morning," she said, "Medifast* Weight Control Center. Can I help you?"

Of course, you can. I've become a fat bastard and I'm through looking like a blimp. I'm round and my health is questionable. I get winded looking at a stairwell—even downward. I strain to push an elevator call button.

Don't worry. I used different words. My call, however, actually was one of desperation. I had failed miserably in my latest attempts to trim down. I needed a jump-start. I was certain I could continue on and change my lifestyle for the better, if I could just drop the first few pounds to get me going.

Advertisements for the diet plan sounded promising. I know all such programs make the same claims—drastic weight loss with little effort. Everyone is (or should be) skeptical. I'm no exception. I know there is no magic pill or formula. In fact, I'm probably tougher on them (advertisers) than most people. Friends and family are tired of hearing me yell at the television.

A local radio personality became a spokeswoman for program after losing more than 100 pounds. I insisted to myself that there probably was more involved than just the diet. Those were fantastic results. Even if this diet plan was only partly responsible, I thought, it was

---

* Medifast is a trademark of Jason Enterprises, Inc., an entity with which the author had no affiliation before, during or following his particpation in the named diet program.

enough to make me consider it.

I found myself on the phone arranging to meet with one of their counselors. "Yes, I'd like to make an appointment to talk to someone about your diet plan," I said. The lovely voice at the other end asked how much weight I needed to lose. "About 40 pounds ought to do it," I replied. They had someone available the day and time I requested.

Their facility was in an office complex where two busy streets intersected. Their unit was tucked away in a corner of the second floor. It was quiet except for the low hum of canned music. The entryway and reception area were neat and clean.

The voice I had encountered was sitting in a chair behind a counter. Her beaming smile made me feel welcome, although there was no way I could be comfortable. I was about to admit to strangers, in person now, that I had been unable to take care of myself. I had let myself go and now I needed help. I felt shame but convinced myself I was being courageous, taking the necessary steps to rectify the situation. I also reminded myself that numerous people had trampled this trail before me and emerged in a happier state of mind and body.

After we briefly exchanged some pleasantries, I sat and flipped through the pages of a scrapbook chock-full of success stories. I had to pry the pages apart at each turn, since the plastic coverings clung to each other. It was as though I was wandering through an old collection of my family photos. These were people I had never seen, however, posing first with a frown then with a smile in before and after pictures. I wondered whether I could equal or surpass their accomplishments. I painted a mental picture of the new me.

My counselor greeted me with her own smile. She took me to an office where we chatted for a few minutes. Her desk was angled to cut across one of the room's corners. One wall was transparent, a row of windows, displaying the streets below. The crossing avenues were filled with cars buzzing this way and that, no doubt hurrying their occupants to the numerous drive-thru restaurant windows that peppered the immediate area.

Her desktop was uninterrupted. A few motivational posters accompanied healthy-food posters on the remaining walls. She sat with her shoulders squared with the floor, her back stretched tall. She seemed a good weight for her height.

Now, about me. Actually, about me in the weight-loss program. She told me the basics—eat the food, shed the pounds—and walked me to meet an apparatus. It looked like half a robot. It had a floor piece with shapes of feet etched upon it. Hmm, what should I put there? The bottom piece hosted a bar that ran upward until it changed angle and split into two poles that extended outward. I pried off my shoes, peeled away my socks, climbed aboard, took hold of the "handle bars," and followed the verbal instructions.

She threw a switch. The machine whirred. She told me to remain motionless while the contraption sized me up. Apparently, it was measuring and analyzing my pulse, posture, and poundage, among other things. The clatter of rollers in a nearby laser printer signaled the end of my encounter with the metallic investigator.

My counselor looked over the provided report and announced that I needed to lose 68 pounds to achieve the proper weight for my height. Yikes! I admitted that I didn't believe that was possible. I knew the charts always recommended I should be that skinny, but it really was unimaginable. I scoffed.

"That's a lofty goal," I said. "I don't believe I can get all the way there, but I admire your ambition." I was quite prepared to have them help me get halfway there. That would be the great jump-start I was hoping to find. I had heard from a friend that

weight loss begins immediately, in the first week. He had participated in this program and thought highly of it.

Then, she shocked me. She said her company guarantees that I will reach my goal weight, if I follow the program without deviation for the specified time frame. "Seriously?" I said. Absolutely, was the response. With that, I figured I couldn't lose. Even if they were wrong, or I failed, I would still lose plenty of weight along the way. So, ready or not, here I...

"I'm going to think about it," I said. "I will let you know in a few days."

That morphed in to a few weeks. I was hesitant, not because I doubted the program. I was unsure of myself. I guess the poor habits and attitude that led me to pack on the fat were keeping me from committing. I was afraid I would miss the food I had come to love, in heaping portions, of course. (That turned out to be true. And I am dang happy about it.)

I engaged in my last episodes of horrendous eating by making several trips to selected restaurants. I gnawed the remains of my junk-food desires. I said goodbye to my favorite eating establishments, at least for a while, and set out to follow the plan created for me by my new partners in fitness and health.

I wished myself luck. But I knew I needed none. I only required determination. And I had plenty.

So, it was with an attitude that I picked up the phone, snapped the receiver to my ear and pounded out the numbers to connect with them again. "I'm ready to sign up and begin the program," I said. They asked me what time I would like to visit.

The office seemed different this time. The music blasting from the ceiling belonged to an annoying genre. Traffic noise from the streets below penetrated the glass barriers. Horns honked. Engines revved. Tires squealed.

Were cold feet causing a greater sensitivity in my ears? I had thought I was nothing but enthused. But, I did experience some awkward moments. The person I had dealt with during my initial visit greeted me and, shortly thereafter, passed me off to another "counselor." And that person heaped information on me, all the details about what I could eat and when. The schooling became very detailed. That is what I had feared.

Simplicity is what had drawn me to this program. I got a bit nervous. I told myself that my reaction was normal for the situation and that the procedures would become very easy very

fast, as soon as a day or two of the routine was behind me. It was too early to make such a judgment.

I was escorted to a food room to make selections from the neatly organized shelves. The plan I would be following called for me to eat five meals per day from the packaged offerings. The sixth I would make at home according to specific instructions. This is where I found the simplicity I sought. Many food packets supposedly would explode into tasty meals with the mere addition of water. Others were a variety of snack bars and drinks. I had been allowed to try a peanut butter bar on my previous visit. It was excellent. I trusted the others would be, too. The only remaining concern was whether the portions would be enough. I convinced myself the answer would be yes. The plan also calls for heaping helpings of water throughout the day. I knew that would help to fill my belly.

Some of the packets are drink mixes. I assumed they would taste good, but one is called a "shake." It is a powder to be churned with water and ice. I was unwilling to toss out an assumption about that quality.

Finally, I was led back to the reception area where I paid for my food selections. That was another awkward moment. There were many people there. Some it seemed already were in the program and visiting for a checkup. Others seemed to be inquiring about starting their own programs.

I felt exposed. I am a bit shy, anyway, but this, to me, was a private situation. I didn't want to share it with other people who were not on the professional side of the coin. I would have preferred to leave through a back door the way psychiatric patients are allowed to depart through a secluded rear exit so they don't have to cross paths with incoming help-seekers—or so I'm told.

It wasn't over, though. They brought me back around the corner and had me pose for pictures, the "before" version. I understood they wanted to have a record of my original form with which to compare after I got rid of all the unwanted body baggage. Still, I was uncomfortable. I grinned and let them have their way with me.

I hope they got my good side. Or, should they have gotten my bad side. That would have been any side. So, I suppose the mission was accomplished. They got my frontal view and turned me to my right. Wait! There was a worse side they could have photographed. I should be thrilled that—to my knowledge—they missed it.

Perhaps they grabbed that angle on my way out. It wouldn't have been a clear view, however. The giant bag of food boxes, measuring cups, instruction booklets, body analysis papers, et al, surely would have been prominent in the picture. Maybe that would be invited. Everything was emblazoned with a colossal and contrasting diet plan logo on it. Good thing I wasn't trying to be discreet.

I said goodbye to the third "counselor" with whom I interacted. She was to be the person I would see on my weekly visits. She also would answer any questions I would have. She would accept emails or phone calls at almost any time. That is a nice benefit.

Aside from feeling a bit sheepish, I was enthused and had a spring in my step as I crossed the parking lot with all my gear, ready to begin my weight loss program… and hide my face from anyone I might encounter before I could duck into my car.

Weights & Measures

*A*ny program to shed unwanted fat should begin with a record of the starting point, not only in weight but in body shape, too. My distorted form had the measurements listed below on the first day of my diet program.

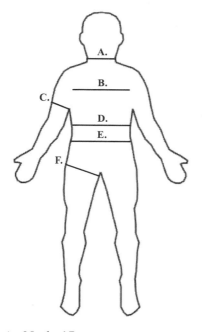

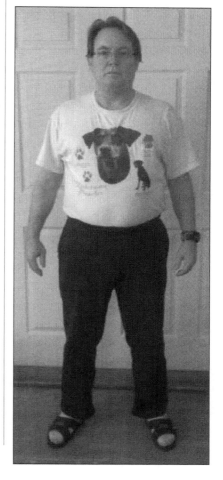

A. Neck: 17

B. Chest: 46

C. Biceps: 13

D. Waist (navel): 45

E. High Hip (belt line): 40

F. Thighs: 25

G. Weight: 207

2

Program launch is no time to be timid

Well, here I go. As I launch into this endeavor, my thoughts are not on whether I will fail... well, not outright. I have a little nervousness over two points: 1) whether the food will be tasty and filling, and 2) whether I will be able to sustain the prescribed eating schedule all the way to the end.

They have set me onto a 34-week program. That is a pretty long time, even if one is not having to work hard for something. I believe I am close to an answer on the first concern. They let me sample a peanut butter bar and it was awesome. If the other food selections are even close to being that good, taste will not be an issue.

I am clueless as to whether meals will be sufficiently filling. That answer will be discovered when the sun sets on my first full day in the program.

I have no idea how long it will take me to have an educated guess on my ability to go the long haul.

What I do know, though, is that I am quite capable of completing things, even difficult ones.

The most important element is determination and I have that in abundance.

9

Day: # *1*   Weight: *207*

Food & Water

7:00 a.m.	cappuccino	2:40 p.m.	3rd water done
9:10 a.m.	cinnamon crunch bar	3:05 p.m.	chocolate shake
9:30 a.m.	pills	6:15 p.m.	4th water done
9:40 a.m.	1st water done	8:00 p.m.	pre-made (p-m) turkey
12:30 p.m.	ziti marinara		meatball marinara
12:45 p.m.	2nd water done		

Exercise

No exercise permitted yet.

Comments

First "meal" was cappuccino. First sip... wow! That actually tastes really good. The cinnamon crunch bar looks tiny. It tastes really good, though. I'll eat it slowly and enjoy. I think I'll get used to the smaller amounts. Drinking water between bites is helping. Water is good and filling.

Almost forgot to take the pills (B-12, super omegas and a probiotic).

My mind has been imagining how I'll look at the end of this program. Cool!

Went to get packaged food replacements for my "normal" meal and some for reserve.

Ziti marinara lunch tasted good. I was afraid it would fail to expand beyond its initial soupy look. It became a bit like chili. I am surprised by how much I enjoyed the chocolate "shake."

First sip... wow!
That actually
tastes really good.

10

Day: #**2**   Weight: **204**

Food & Water

7:10 a.m.	cappuccino
7:30 a.m.	pills
9:30 a.m.	cinnamon crunch bar
9:40 a.m.	1st water done
12:15 p.m.	ziti marinara
1:15 p.m.	2nd water done

3:30 p.m.	chocolate shake
5:30 p.m.	3rd water
8:00 p.m.	(p-m) chicken, rice, vegetables
8:15 p.m.	brownie

Exercise

No exercise permitted yet.

Comments

My weigh-in this morning showed me three pounds lighter than yesterday. I am unsure what to make of it. I would say it is merely water loss, but I have been hydrating plenty, maybe even in excess. Anyway, I am sure it will balance out.

Regardless, it is a step in the right direction.

Today I realized that I have no lust for bad (processed) food. That's a good thing. The pre-made "normal" meals are a great option. They require no mixing or measuring. Just peel back a corner of the wrapper and microwave for 90 seconds.

> *Today I realized that I have no lust for bad (processed) food.*

Day: #3   Weight: *202.*⁴

Food & Water

7:30 a.m.	cappuccino		3:35 p.m.	peanut butter bar
9:30 a.m.	cinnamon crunch bar		4:45 p.m.	4th water done
9:40 a.m.	1st water done		7:45 p.m.	(p-m) beef stew
9:45 a.m.	pills (1st B-12)		8:10 p.m.	brownie
11:30 a.m.	2nd water done		8:15 p.m.	5th water
12:45 p.m.	ziti marinara		8:30 p.m.	pill (2nd B-12)
3:30 p.m.	3rd water done			

Exercise

No exercise permitted yet.

Comments

Feeling a little weak this morning, I thought for a moment that I might just be tired. But I know I got seven hours of sleep last night. So, that shouldn't be it.

I'm looking forward to my morning cappuccino and some cold water to follow.

I'm at work now and no longer feeling weakness. Excellent! And that's not the cappuccino talking. I haven't had it yet.

Went to the employee lounge to get ice for my water bottle and there was a platter of free pastries. I laughed at it, having zero interest. I would have stuffed myself just a few days ago. My only second thought was one of amazement of how uninterested I was in eating that. I am thrilled to have such willpower. And it's been basically effortless.

Feeling energetic. I just brushed off the elevator and took the stairs—three floors. Okay, I was going down, but that's a start.

I swapped in a peanut butter crunch bar for my "usual" shake in the afternoon. Boy, those are good.

Day: #4   Weight: 201.²

Food & Water

7:30 a.m.	cappuccino	3:10 p.m.	4th water done
9:30 a.m.	cinnamon crunch bar	3:30 p.m.	peanut butter bar
9:40 a.m.	1st water done	5:10 p.m.	pill (2nd B-12)
10:40 a.m.	2nd water done	7:30 p.m.	(p-m) chicken
12:30 p.m.	3rd water done		cacciatore
12:45 p.m.	chili	8:30 p.m.	5th water done
1:30 p.m.	pills	10:00 p.m.	brownie

Exercise

No exercise permitted yet.

Comments

I got an email from my program counselor. She cheerfully encouraged me and noted that I was experiencing ketosis (abnormal fat metabolism). Ah, my old friend. We meet again.

Last time was when I did the no-carbohydrate Atkins diet. This program, however, gives me the right carbs, so I have no pain in my kidneys. I'm quite glad of that.

She also said I should be feeling more energetic with a loss of appetite. Well, no, I feel a little run down and, although my scale says I'm losing weight, my legs feel a little heavier (read weak).

I went to the employee lounge to fill my water bottle with ice and found someone had brought cupcakes and cookies to share. It's a common occurrence. Often, it's donuts. This company could never starve.

I was uninterested. I walked away clean. My only thought was to get a camera and return for a picture. Did it. Still no interest in eating those things. That's a big change, though. Last week I would have gobbled three cupcakes and a couple of cookies.

I am convinced bad food creates a desire for more.

13

Day: #*5*   Weight: *199.*⁸

Food & Water

9:00 a.m.	cappuccino	4:00 p.m.	4th water done
10:15 a.m.	1st water done	4:30 p.m.	peanut butter bar
11:30 a.m.	cinnamon crunch bar	5:30 p.m.	5th water
11:45 a.m.	2nd water done	7:30 p.m.	(p-m) turkey meatball marinara
1:45 p.m.	3rd water done		
2:15 p.m.	chili	8:20 p.m.	6th water
2:20 p.m.	pills (1st B-12)	9:40 p.m.	peanut butter soft serve

Exercise

No exercise permitted yet.

Comments

Took the kids to McDonald's as usual on a Saturday to let them abuse the play room. I am happy to report that I had no interest in ordering food from the menu for myself.

I also got away having spent half the usual fare. Saving money is good, too.

I am happy to report I had no interest in ordering food from the menu for myself.

14

Day: #*6*   Weight: **200.**²

Food & Water

9:00 a.m.	cappuccino	7:20 p.m.	pills (first B-12)
11:30 a.m.	cinnamon crunch bar	7:35 p.m.	chicken, rice, veggies
2:00 p.m.	1st water done		(p-m)
2:30 p.m.	chili	7:40 p.m.	3rd water done
4:30 p.m.	peanut butter bar	9:30 p.m.	brownie
4:35 p.m.	2nd water done	9:40 p.m.	4th water done

Exercise

No exercise permitted yet.

Comments

My weight bounced up a half pound this morning. I am sure I should have expected it. This is a long-term program and the overall result is what counts.

But the feeling is not good. It seems like an unnecessary delay in descent. I am putting in plenty of effort (meals timing, etc.) and want to see steady results. I won't let it stop me, but I much rather would have seen a tiny drop or status quo than a jump upward.

It makes me want even more to be able to exercise. But they won't let me yet!

Having doubts today. I thought of the numerous weeks I will be on the same eating schedule. I thought of an awesome meal. Its image floated in my brain and made me fantasize about eating it.

I am sure it will be fine. In fact, the doubt passed not long after it arrived. I am about to eat, so I figure it is a result of my hunger.

❝

Having doubts today.

❞

15

Day: #*7*   Weight: ***200.*²**

Food & Water

8:15 a.m.	cappuccino	3:25 p.m.	pill (2nd B-12)
10:30 a.m.	1st water done	4:00 p.m.	peanut butter bar
10:45 a.m.	cinnamon crunch bar	6:30 p.m.	4th water done
11:30 a.m.	2nd water done	7:30 p.m.	chicken, broccoli
1:05 p.m.	pills (1st B-12)	7:40 p.m.	5th water done
1:30 p.m.	chili	10:30 p.m.	brownie
2:30 p.m.	3rd water done		

Exercise

No exercise permitted yet.

Comments

I am frustrated by having the same weight this morning as I did yesterday! It doesn't mean I will quit. That is not an option.

But I would like to see continued and steady progress.

Today I ate my first "normal" meal. I had been eating the "pre-made" stand-in meals.

They are okay, but wow! Tonight I ate six ounces of chicken and one-and-a-half cups of broccoli. That was a real meal.

The chicken was a "slab" worthy of worship. The broccoli was about the amount I would eat at a "normal" pre-diet meal.

This meal was way more filling than a packaged meal on the plan. It was awesome.

I could get used to this type of eating.

I could get used to this type of eating.

16

AFTER ONE WEEK

IMPRESSIONS & PROGRESS

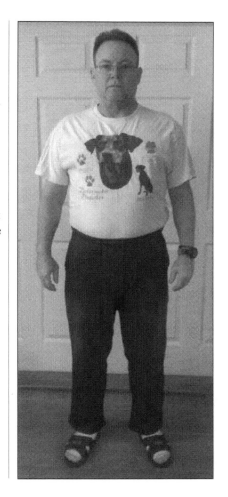

Well, I have a full week of the program—pardon the pun—under my belt. The first thing I noticed was that the small-looking food portions actually turned out to be sufficiently filling. Eating slowly helped, too.

The second is that, almost immediately, I lost my appetite for bad food. Also, the "normal" meal is awesome. It's not only a home-cooked meal; the protein item and vegetables taste excellent and can remain in my diet after the program ends.

My only craving, really, was for exercise. I know I would much enjoy lifting some weights and swimming or running. It is prohibited, however, this early in the schedule.

In summary, I have no regrets. I am happy to be in the program. I have seen good results so far and I am excited about knocking off more poundage.

Day: #*8*   Weight: *199.*²

Food & Water

8:15 a.m.	cappuccino	5:15 p.m.	4th water done
8:30 a.m.	pills (1st B-12)	8:10 p.m.	talapia (fish), broccoli
9:00 a.m.	1st water done	8:20 p.m.	5th water
10:10 a.m.	2nd water done	10:30 p.m.	brownie
11:30 a.m.	cinnamon crunch bar		
2:15 p.m.	peanut butter bar		
2:30 p.m.	3rd water done		

Exercise

No exercise permitted yet.

Comments

Yeehaw! I'm back down a pound from yesterday. It is good to be dropping weight again.

Today is the day of my first weekly visit to the program office for evaluation.

My counselor said I was doing well and appreciated the extra detail I provided in my daily log book.

I had a weigh-in and measurements taken but not a scan from the robot to analyze my body, as was performed before I began the program. That function will be accomplished every two weeks.

The talapia and broccoli dinner I ate was excellent. I'm still impressed that the weight and size of the fish is quite sufficient.

It is good to be dropping weight again.

Day: #*9*   Weight: *199.⁰*

Food & Water

8:00 a.m.	cappuccino	4:00 p.m.	cinnamon crunch bar
10:30 a.m.	peanut butter bar	6:30 p.m.	4th water done
11:15 a.m.	1st water done	7:30 p.m.	pill (2nd B-12)
11:30 a.m.	pills (1st B-12)	7:45 p.m.	ground turkey,
1:40 p.m.	2nd water done		broccoli, asparagus
1:45 p.m.	chili	8:00 p.m.	5th water done
3:30 p.m.	3rd water done		

Exercise

No exercise permitted yet.

Comments

I went out and about today and realized that a person who lives life on the go may find it slightly inconvenient to keep this eating schedule.

I have what is characterized as a desk job. I don't have to abandon the office too often. That allows me to eat or drink on cue.

Today, however, I'm on vacation (at home) and found myself wandering the maze at Ikea with a cinnamon crunch bar in my hand.

I had to carry it with me because the bewitching (meal) hour was going to strike while I was away from the house. I couldn't leave it in the car, lest it melt to a gooey blob in the heat.

Still, this is a minor inconvenience. A little planning, and maybe an ice chest, would make it all go pretty well.

...a person who lives life on the go may find it slightly inconvenient to keep this eating schedule.

Day: # *10*   Weight: *198.⁸*

Food & Water

8:45 a.m.	cappuccino
9:00 a.m.	pills (1st B-12)
10:45 a.m.	cinnamon crunch bar
11:10 a.m.	1st water done
1:00 p.m.	2nd water done
1:30 p.m.	chili
4:15 p.m.	peanut butter bar

4:30 p.m.	3rd water done
6:45 p.m.	4th water done
7:45 p.m.	ground turkey, broccoli
8:00 p.m.	5th water done
10:30 p.m.	chocolate shake
10:45 p.m.	6th water

Exercise

No exercise permitted yet.

Comments

I was so busy; I had a little difficulty remembering to eat.

I was on the go today, taking the kids to school and working around the house. I hung blinds on five windows and watched my wife build an Ikea computer desk.

I was so busy; I had a little difficulty remembering to eat. I kept fairly close to the schedule, but I think all the work was a lot like exercise—which I am supposed to be avoiding.

It was good to strain, but that may have been why I was extra hungry by the time we sat down to dinner, me to my "normal" meal of ground turkey and broccoli. It tasted great.

20

Day: # *11*   Weight: *198.*⁶

Food & Water

8:00 a.m.	cappuccino	4:30 p.m.	peanut butter bar
8:45 a.m.	pills (1st B-12)	6:00 p.m.	4th water done
10:25 a.m.	cinnamon crunch bar	7:00 p.m.	ground turkey,
10:30 a.m.	1st water done		broccoli, asparagus
1:15 p.m.	2nd water done	9:00 p.m.	5th water done
1:30 p.m.	ziti marinara	10:00 p.m.	peanut butter bar
4:00 p.m.	3rd water done		

Exercise

No exercise permitted yet.

Comments

This morning's weigh-in only showed two-tenths of a pound reduction from yesterday. I have come to expect more. The fault may be on my positioning of the scale in regard to a floor mat in my bathroom. I will be very particular about that in the future to avoid any doubts.

I have come to expect more.

21

Day: # *12*   Weight: *197.*⁶

Food & Water

9:15 a.m.	cappuccino
9:30 a.m.	pills (1st B-12)
11:00 a.m.	1st water done
11:45 a.m.	peanut butter bar
3:00 p.m.	chili
3:15 p.m.	pill (2nd B-12)
5:45 p.m.	cinnamon crunch bar

6:30 p.m.	2nd water done
8:45 p.m.	chicken, cauliflower, asparagus
10:00 p.m.	3rd water done
10:45 p.m.	peanut butter soft serve
11:00 p.m.	4th water done

Exercise

No exercise permitted yet.

Comments

I had been having some low-level pain in my stomach. I was going to email my program counselor, if it continued, but I think I figured it out.

I was out and about today and finished my first water on the road. After a few hours, even though I was reaching the three-hour mark without food, I was feeling fine. I had thought the discomfort was caused by hunger. Now I think that too much water might have been causing the bad feeling. I will keep a close eye on my liquid intake and see how it goes. I will try drinking only the amount recommended, rather than exceeding it, as I have been, and see what happens. I also am going to send that message to confirm with my program contact.

Now I think that too much water might have been causing the bad feeling.

22

Day: #13   Weight: 197.⁶

Food & Water

8:30 a.m.	cappuccino
8:45 a.m.	pills (1st B-12)
11:15 a.m.	cinnamon bar
11:30 a.m.	1st water done
2:15 p.m.	ziti marinara
2:30 p.m.	pill (2nd B-12)
4:15 p.m.	2nd water done
5:00 p.m.	peanut butter bar
7:45 p.m.	3rd water done
8:00 p.m.	talapia, lettuce, broccoli
9:30 p.m.	peanut butter soft serve

Exercise

No exercise permitted yet.

Comments

Drat! My weight is the same as yesterday. Well, as I noted before, these plateaus are expected. They sure don't feel good, though.

When you are very strict in adherence to the plan, you expect some tangible result. When you do your part, you expect the weight gods to do theirs. Of course, it doesn't always work out that way.

I kept my water intake to about the required 64 ounces and didn't experience any stomach discomfort. I am pretty glad to have that issue under control.

When you do your part, you expect the weight gods to do theirs.

23

Day: #**14**   Weight: **197.²**

Food & Water

7:30 a.m.	cappuccino		6:30 p.m.	3rd water done
10:30 a.m.	peanut butter bar		8:00 p.m.	ground turkey, broccoli
11:15 a.m.	1st water done			
1:30 p.m.	ziti marinara		8:20 p.m.	pill (2nd B-12)
3:00 p.m.	2nd water done		9:30 p.m.	chocolate shake
4:30 p.m.	chocolate shake			
4:35 p.m.	pills (1st B-12)			

Exercise

No exercise permitted yet

Comments

That tends to make me describe this diet (process) as EASY!

Donuts and cookies in the employee lounge! AGAIN! Fortunately, I had no interest in sampling any of those sugary disasters.

That tends to make me describe this diet (process) as EASY! I am having absolutely no struggles with hunger.

I have a late entry for "pills" because I almost forgot. All I had to do was take them out of my bag and swallow them. They slipped my mind until I got home from work and unloaded my gear.

Another day of drinking close to the needed amount of water and my stomach is still good.

24

AFTER TWO WEEKS

IMPRESSIONS & PROGRESS

I "groped the robot" (got analyzed by company hardware) on this week's visit to the program office.

It said I dropped 10 pounds in my first 14 days! But not only fat is being banished. I have lost some muscle. My counselor said to add three ounces of protein to my "normal" meal.

I am feeling pretty good, still no hunger. I eat at regular intervals and enjoy the tastes. My clothes are getting loose and I am more comfortable wearing them. I am looking forward to purchasing new attire for the new me.

My only frustration (minimal) is that on a couple of occasions my weight bounced up slightly. I could avoid the feeling that goes with these slumps by only weighing in once per week. That is not possible, though, as I am too excited about the journey and need to monitor my progress closely. I will just have to deal with it and stay focused for the long haul to a fit, trim and healthy body.

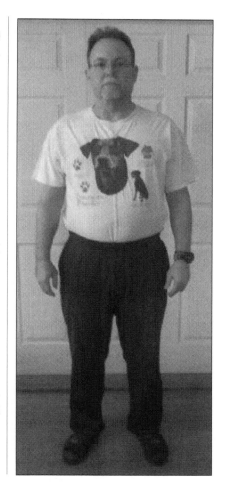

Day: #*15*   Weight: *197.⁰*

Food & Water

7:10 a.m.	chocolate shake	4:45 p.m.	pill (2nd B-12)
7:25 a.m.	pills (1st B-12)	5:00 p.m.	2nd water done
9:15 a.m.	brownie	8:00 p.m.	talapia, broccoli, asparagus
11:30 a.m.	1st water done	9:15 p.m.	3rd water done
1:15 p.m.	ziti marinara	10:00 p.m.	peanut butter soft serve
4:30 p.m.	peanut butter soft serve		

Exercise

I have been given the green light to exercise and, as much as I have been longing to get going, work kept me from a workout today.

Comments

This morning I had to make some clothing adjustments because my pants were too loose to wear to work.

That's the kind of change I like to see. I won't mind if I have to buy a complete new wardrobe at the end of this program.

I am more comfortable in my clothes and I feel lighter and smaller.

I had to wrench my belt up a notch as a result of my first two weeks of the program. And that is without exercise.

I am pleased.

I had to wrench my belt up a notch as a result of my first two weeks of the program. And that is without exercise.

Day: # *16*   Weight: *197.*⁴

Food & Water

8:00 a.m.   cappuccino
11:00 a.m. pills (1st B-12)
11:15 a.m. cinnamon bar
1:00 p.m.   1st water done
1:30 p.m.   chili
4:30 p.m.   peanut butter bar
5:30 p.m.   pill (2nd B-12)

6:30 p.m.   2nd water done
8:00 p.m.   ground turkey,
            broccoli
10:30 p.m. 3rd water done
11:00 p.m. chocolate pudding

Exercise

None today.

Comments

Well, my weigh-in this morning showed my weight bounced up two-tenths of a pound. I have no idea why, but it makes me want to exercise even more.

I will try to get a short run in tonight. That should make me feel better, if not physically, then mentally.

I want to feel like I am doing more to achieve my goal, something other than just eating certain things at specific times.

By the time I went to bed, however, my run remained elusive.

I want to feel like I am doing more to achieve my goal, something other than just eating certain things at specific times.

27

Day: # *17*   Weight: *195.*⁸

Food & Water

7:00 a.m.	cappuccino		4:00 p.m.	peanut butter bar
7:20 a.m.	pills (1st B-12)		7:30 p.m.	3rd water done
10:00 a.m.	cinnamon bar		8:00 p.m.	chicken, broccoli,
10:05 a.m.	1st water done			asparagus
1:00 p.m.	chili		10:00 p.m.	4th water done
1:30 p.m.	pill (2nd B-12)		10:15 p.m.	nacho cheese puffs
3:15 p.m.	2nd water done			

Exercise

Swim: 20 laps, 30 minutes.

Comments

I awoke this morning in fear of my scale. The previous bump worried me. It was for nothing, however. My weight was down almost a pound-and-a-half. Just as I should not be gloomy about a jump, I should not get too excited about this "achievement."

I reminded myself that it is a long process. Tomorrow the number may rise. I have got to acknowledge that progress is being made.

I went swimming today. It felt great to get back into the water. I kept my pace easy. I figured I shouldn't work too hard on my first day back. There will be plenty of time to push my

> *I awoke this morning in fear of the scale.*

body. Still, a while after and into the night, I was pretty beat. I'm not sure if it was more water and sun that got me or the actual exertion. Regardless, I will sleep well tonight and dream about the morning bout with my scale.

28

Day: #**18**   Weight: **196.**^{0}

Food & Water

7:30 a.m.	cappuccino
9:00 a.m.	pills (1st B-12)
10:30 a.m.	cinnamon bar
1:30 p.m.	chili
2:00 p.m.	1st water done
2:10 p.m.	pill (2nd B-12)
4:30 p.m.	peanut butter bar

5:00 p.m.	2nd water done
7:00 p.m.	turkey, broccoli
8:00 p.m.	3rd water done
10:30 p.m.	chocolate pudding

Exercise

No exercise today.

Comments

...yesterday's significant drop (in weight) serves as quite a cushion for me to accept today's hiccup.

As suspected, my weight jumped a smidgen. It was up two-tenths of a pound this morning at weigh-in. But yesterday's significant drop serves as quite a cushion for me to accept today's hiccup.

So, I will press on, eating as scheduled and enjoying the tastes, knowing the process is still working.

A note on taste, since I brought it up: I am not a fan of the nacho cheese puffs. They were unexpectedly dry and spicy. They are like a hard crunch, too, like croutons in a salad. They are not for me.

Day: #*19*   Weight: *195.*²

Food & Water

9:00 a.m.   cappuccino
9:15 a.m.   pills (1st B-12)
11:30 a.m. 1st water done
12:00 p.m. cinnamon bar
2:00 p.m.   2nd water done
3:00 p.m.   chili
3:30 p.m.   pill (2nd B-12)

6:00 p.m.   peanut butter bar
6:05 p.m.   3rd water done
9:00 p.m.   turkey, zucchini
11:00 p.m. peanut butter soft
            serve

Exercise

Run: 15 minutes.

Comments

It will get easier as the days pass-- guaranteed.

My weigh-in showed the downward trend again. Good thing I didn't get excited about yesterday's bump.

I took my first run of the program this morning. Running is good, hard work. It was especially so today. My legs hurt a lot. It wasn't because of my breathing, etc. The culprit was my excessive weight. It will get easier as the days pass—guaranteed.

Day: #*20*   Weight: *195.⁰*

Food & Water

8:30 a.m.	cappuccino
12:00 p.m.	cinnamon bar
12:10 p.m.	1st water done
2:30 p.m.	chili
3:00 p.m.	2nd water done
5:00 p.m.	peanut butter bar
7:00 p.m.	3rd water done

8:00 p.m.	beef, turkey, broccoli
8:30 p.m.	pills (1st B-12)
10:15 p.m.	peanut butter soft serve
10:30 p.m.	pill (2nd B-12)

Exercise

Run: 15 minutes; Jumping jacks, 100; Weights: bench press, 100 lbs., 1 set of 10 reps; curls, 20 lbs., 1 set of 10 reps each arm

Comments

Running was a bit easier and a lot more fun this morning. My son asked if he could exercise with me today. He and his sister joined me in stretching and a circle of the neighborhood. After that, we did jumping jacks. The twin six-year-olds continued with push-ups and sit-ups, making them great role models for their old man. I aspire to be more like them in many other ways, too.

An interesting note: my workout (and water consumption) today made me completely forget about food. I had a brain lapse and was a little late for my eating appointment.

...my workout (and water consumption) today made me completely forget about food.

31

Day: #**21**   Weight: **193.**^*8*

Food & Water

8:00 a.m.	cappuccino
9:45 a.m.	pills (1st B-12)
10:30 a.m.	cinnamon bar
1:30 p.m.	chili
2:00 p.m.	pill (2nd B-12)
2:30 p.m.	1st water done
4:30 p.m.	peanut butter bar

7:30 p.m.	turkey, broccoli, asparagus
8:00 p.m.	2nd water done
10:00 p.m.	chocolate pudding
11:00 p.m.	3rd water done

Exercise

None today.

Comments

Wow! Another pleasant (sizable) drop in weight this morning. I know it will balance out, but it still feels good. I also wonder if I may have just burned many more calories than usual because I had such a great day of exercise and work around the house.

Well, I will know more at tomorrow's rendezvous with the scale.

Since I was directed to eat extra protein, I added the necessary portion to tonight's meal. Ten ounces of 99% fat-free ground turkey was too much to eat. I guess my stomach has shrunk a lot.

Wow! Another sizable drop in weight this morning. I know it will balance out, but it still feels good.

AFTER THREE WEEKS

IMPRESSIONS & PROGRESS

It is a bit odd. I haven't exactly had cravings, but I have had a few of my old favorite meals pop into my head and make me feel a bit interested in them. I suppose that sounds an awful lot like a craving. The difference is that the images existed without any accompanying urges to eat.

So, the occurrences will not create an issue or nudge me from my course. It just has been interesting seeing some of my old restaurant favorites "floating" through my thoughts.

In this diet program, eating out is not specifically prohibited. The counselors provide each participant with a pocket-size menu guide to make the right food choices when a dieter, for whatever reason, suddenly finds himself in a restaurant at meal time. There are ways to partake in the offerings without exceeding the program's limitations on food types and quantities.

So there need be no heavy guilt.

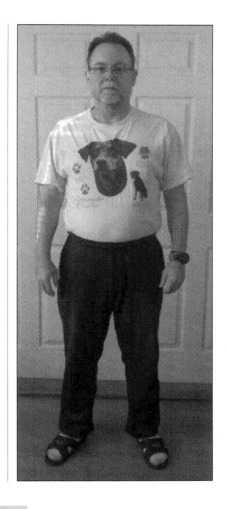

Day: #*22*   Weight: *194.*[8]

Food & Water

8:00 a.m.	cappuccino	5:00 p.m.	pill (2nd B-12)
10:15 a.m.	cinnamon bar	5:30 p.m.	2nd water done
11:20 a.m.	pills (1st B-12)	7:30 p.m.	turkey, broccoli
1:15 p.m.	chili	8:00 p.m.	3rd water done
2:00 p.m.	1st water done	10:15 p.m.	apple cinnamon
3:00 p.m.	chili		oatmeal
4:15 p.m.	peanut butter bar		

Exercise

None today.

Comments

I told ya so! I witnessed another bounce this morning. This one was a full pound. I won't let it get me down. I must continue plugging away and keep an eye on the scale.

I am positive it will continue to average out to about two-tenths of a pound per day. That seems to be on track to make my goal weight in the time allotted.

I tried oatmeal for the first time today. It was apple cinnamon flavor and I can see myself eating oatmeal for a long time, since it apparently is good for the body, beyond a weight-loss diet.

I won't let it get me down. I must continue plugging away and keep an eye on the scale.

34

Day: #23   Weight: *193.⁰*

Food & Water

7:30 a.m.	cappuccino	4:00 p.m.	lemon meringue bar
10:00 a.m.	fruit & nut bar	5:00 p.m.	2nd water done
10:30 a.m.	pills (1st B-12)	7:00 p.m.	talapia, broccoli
11:00 a.m.	1st water done	10:15 p.m.	brownie
1:00 p.m.	macaroni & cheese, turkey	11:00 p.m.	3rd water done
1:30 p.m.	pill (2nd B-12)		

Exercise

Swim: 20 laps, 27 minutes.

Comments

I had another significant drop in weight this morning. It was more than a pound, but I am able to ignore it. I just tell myself to think of the day's work ahead and carry on.

My swim today was enjoyable. (Can a swim be unpleasant?) I even improved my time a bit without pushing myself. I am still taking it fairly easy.

I am going slowly not only because I have fewer calories to fuel me but also because exercise and I have become strangers over the last couple of years.

It would be wise, I think, to get reacquainted with a patient approach.

My swim today was enjoyable (Can a swim be unpleasant?) I even improved my time a bit without pushing myself.

Day: #**24**   Weight: **194.**⁰

Food & Water

7:30 a.m.	cappuccino		4:30 p.m.	pill (2nd B-12)
9:15 a.m.	pills (1st B-12)		8:00 p.m.	pork chop, broccoli
10:15 a.m.	fruit & nut bar		8:30 p.m.	2nd water done
1:15 p.m.	macaroni & cheese		9:30 p.m.	apple cinnamon
3:00 p.m.	1st water done			oatmeal
3:00 p.m.	chili		11:00 p.m.	3rd water done
4:15 p.m.	lemon meringue bar			

Exercise

None today.

Comments

I felt some hunger while I was juggling tasks. It made me think the stress I was experiencing was burning extra calories.

My weight jumped a full pound. I guess the tracking trend would look like the teeth on a tree saw. I must ignore it and continue with the plan, knowing it will be on the down slope tomorrow.

My job got really hectic today with a major project and imminent deadline. I felt some hunger while I was juggling tasks. It made me think that the stress I was experiencing was burning extra calories. I guess that is the only benefit of the pressures of employment.

36

Day: #*25*   Weight: *192.⁸*

Food & Water

7:15 a.m.	cappuccino	4:30 p.m.	lemon meringue bar
9:30 a.m.	pills (1st B-12)	7:30 p.m.	turkey, broccoli
10:30 a.m.	fruit & nut bar	8:00 p.m.	3rd water done
11:00 a.m.	1st water done	10:00 p.m.	brownie
1:30 p.m.	macaroni & cheese		
2:30 p.m.	pill (2nd B-12)		
2:40 p.m.	2nd water done		

Exercise

None today.

Comments

I am feeling quite normal today, as all previous days. It just reminds me that this is a pretty easy routine.

Work is keeping me busy. I also had a good chuckle in the employee lounge. As I entered, the first thing I saw was a display of donuts, two boxes of brightly colored fat pills.

I scooted past, filled my bottle with ice and happily snickered on my way out.

My clothes are fitting much more loosely these days (I am happy to say), but I have not quite shrunk out of them yet.

That will be a great milestone.

My clothes are fitting much more loosely these days... but I have not quite shrunk out of them yet.

Day: #**26**   Weight: **192.**^{0}

Food & Water

8:00 a.m.	apple cinnamon oatmeal
8:05 a.m.	pills (1st B-12)
9:15 a.m.	1st water done
11:00 a.m.	lemon meringue bar
12:30 p.m.	pill (2nd B-12)
2:00 p.m.	fruit & nut bar

4:30 p.m.	2nd water done
5:15 p.m.	macaroni & cheese
8:30 p.m.	turkey, broccoli
9:00 p.m.	3rd water done
9:30 p.m.	brownie

Exercise

None today.

Comments

This afternoon I felt pretty tired, not weak but sleepy. I am supposed to be on the alert for a feeling of extra energy or, the opposite, notable weakness.

I believe my experience today falls outside of those warned-of situations. I may ask my counselor anyway. My meeting with her is just a couple of days away. If I feel overly sleepy tomorrow, I'll email an inquiry rather than wait until my scheduled visit.

I believe my experience today falls outside of those warned-of situations.

Day: #**27**   Weight: **191.**⁴

Food & Water

8:30 a.m.	cappuccino
9:00 a.m.	pills (1st B-12)
10:15 a.m.	1st water done
11:30 a.m.	fruit & nut bar
11:45 a.m.	2nd water done
2:15 p.m.	lemon meringue bar
3:00 p.m.	3rd water done

5:05 p.m.	chocolate shake
5:10 p.m.	pill (2nd B-12)
7:30 p.m.	talapia, broccoli
10:30 p.m.	brownie

Exercise

Run: 25 minutes.
Weights: bench press, squats, curls (bar), curls (dumbbells).

Comments

I woke up okay. The weigh-in was good again. Stretching and running was good work, too. I did have a moment during warm-up when I realized I was just about to hit the one-month mark in this program.

That made me look ahead and see that another 30 weeks remained. That is a long time, I thought. Admittedly, it is. But I can make it. It has been easy so far.

I have adjusted and all is well. There is no turning back. I also fuel my enthusiasm by creating mental images of myself all trimmed down to proper weight.

I also know that, when I am

> *I also fuel my enthusiasm by creating mental images of myself all trimmed down to proper weight.*

that light, I will be able to run in organized competitions. I don't care about winning (I know I will not), but the events will be fun.

Day: #*28*   Weight: *192.⁴*

Food & Water

7:15 a.m.	cappuccino
9:30 a.m.	pills (1st B-12)
10:15 a.m.	fruit & nut bar
10:45 a.m.	1st water done
1:15 p.m.	macaroni & cheese
1:30 p.m.	pill (2nd B-12)
4:00 p.m.	lemon meringue bar

7:00 p.m.	chicken, broccoli, asparagus
7:30 p.m.	2nd water done
10:00 p.m.	apple cinnamon oatmeal
10:30 p.m.	3rd water done

Exercise

None today.

Comments

I had an odd dream last night. The pertinent part was that I departed from my scheduled program and ate French fries. It was peculiar because I knew at the time that I was not supposed to eat them. I believe I felt a moment of regret but knew it was done and the clock couldn't be turned back.

The dream was freakish for another reason. If I were to consider messing up my work in this program, I certainly never would cheat with French fries. I am not their biggest fan. There are so many other delectable meals that would be far more tempting.

Still, I will not budge.

The dream was freakish for another reason... I certainly never would cheat with French fries.

AFTER FOUR WEEKS

IMPRESSIONS & PROGRESS

I noted previously that I think the overall pace I will see in the program is about two-tenths of a pound per day.

I based that on the bouncing I have seen in scale readings. This is the end of four weeks, however, and I have shed roughly 15 pounds, just under four pounds per week.

That is good results. If I could continue that speed until I get where I am going, I would be thrilled. I imagine my counselor will try to slow me down a bit, though, for health reasons.

If there is no danger and I can continue, I will keep working hard and cut my time-to-goal.

In my scheduled visit today, my counselor confirmed my weight loss. She also told me that the long-term average is about two or three pounds per week. So, my almost four is unimpressive and the pace is expected to slow slightly. Okay, I will relax and get back to work.

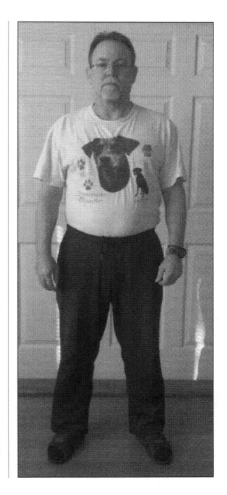

3

The 'robot' is my good friend in loss

Several questions have found clear answers in these first 30 days. In summary, the food is excellent. The amount is adequate. Sticking to the eating schedule is amazingly easy. Finally, I have no doubt I can go the distance and achieve near miraculous weight loss.

The last one is of the utmost importance. I think that, if I were lacking a high level of confidence, I would have to fight not only the demons of fat but also my own mind.

That would be a recipe for almost certain disaster. Fortunately, that is not the case.

I must admit that I am notably impressed by the body analysis machine the folks at the diet company have. I call it the "robot," but it is an awesome helper undeserving of my silly moniker.

It operates thusly. The overweight schlep (me) removes his shoes and socks (they provide a moist towelette to wipe your bare feet) and steps onto the platform, placing heels and toes in designated spots.

The schlep grabs onto two bars that swing up to about waist level. The schlep's thumbs naturally align atop sensors that pass low-intensity electronic pulses into the schlep's body.

As the pulses return to their source, the robot analyzes them and feeds them to a nearby printer.

The counselor glances over the data and reports how many calories the schlep's body will burn in a full day at rest.

It also tells what percentage of the body is muscle, how much is fat and, of course, the overall weight.

These figures are extremely important, especially the muscle content factor. The more muscle the schlep possesses, the more efficiently and quickly the schlep's body will devour calories.

Monitoring the muscle content during the weight-loss process tells the counselor whether muscle is being burned along with unwanted fat.

That is bad. That is what I experienced. My counselor advised me to increase my protein intake to combat that anomaly.

I went even better. My additional exercise actually increased my muscle mass.

That is good.

That brings me to another important consideration: mental attitude. Yes, you need to bring one with you. Having a good report from the robot, however, will put a spring in your step and thrust you happily along the days ahead.

A good report, obviously, results from sticking to the program.

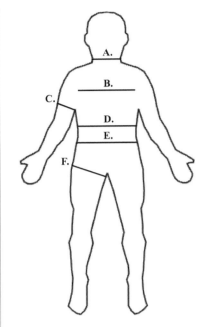

A. Neck: 16.[5]

B. Chest: 45

C. Biceps: 13

D. Waist (navel): 43

E. High Hip (belt line): 39

F. Thighs: 23

G. Weight: 192.[4]

So it is a circle of work and reward.

So, to summarize and conclude my impressions of my first whole month of this diet program, I will say that diligently following the plan should almost guarantee success. At least that is what I am sure of at this moment.

My situation is not all bright and cheerful, however. I saw my reflection in a store-front window and was utterly disgusted. This happened within the last few days.

My horrendous belly reminded me that I have a long journey ahead.

That is okay, though. I am up to the challenge. I also will continue to look at the steady progress I am making and let that be my motivation.

There is, and will be, no instant gratification in a pursuit this important. I will remain conscious that my success will not be measured only by the number of pounds that I drop but by my ability to adopt a new lifestyle, one that includes smart eating and regular exercise.

Day: #*29*   Weight: *191.*^{8}

Food & Water

7:15 a.m.	cappuccino
7:30 a.m.	pills (1st B-12)
10:15 a.m.	fruit & nut bar
11:45 a.m.	1st water done
1:30 p.m.	macaroni & cheese, turkey
2:00 p.m.	pill (2nd B-12)
4:30 p.m.	lemon meringue bar
6:00 p.m.	2nd water done
7:30 p.m.	cod, broccoli
10:00 p.m.	maple, brown sugar oatmeal
10:20 p.m.	3rd water done

Exercise

Swim: 20 laps, 25 minutes.

Comments

The good news is that, not only is my weight continuing to drop, my muscle mass is increasing.

Today was my day to "grope the robot" again. What a machine that is! The good news is that, not only is my weight continuing to drop, my muscle mass is increasing.

The added muscle will help burn fat calories faster. My daily "static" use of energy has risen.

I can burn more than 1,500 calories per day doing nothing. With continued exercise, I can increase the fat burn by far.

Day: #*30*   Weight: *192.²*

Food & Water

7:30 a.m.	cappuccino		7:30 p.m.	talapia, cauliflower, broccoli
8:30 a.m.	pills (1st B-12)			
10:30 a.m.	cinnamon crunch bar		9:30 p.m.	maple, brown sugar oatmeal
11:30 a.m.	1st water done			
2:00 p.m.	pill (2nd B-12)		10:00 p.m.	3rd water done
4:15 p.m.	sloppy joe			
6:00 p.m.	2nd water done			

Exercise

None today.

Comments

Well, I guess it is time to admit that these small upticks in my weight really do bother me. I tried hard to fight it.

So, what is the best way to deal with this? I need to figure it out because it probably will continue throughout the program.

I suppose a good strategy would be to focus my thoughts on another matter. Food, for example, might work.

Today I tried the vegetarian Sloppy Joe. It is slightly spicy with a great taste.

Another significant point is that it seems like real meat. I am looking forward to the next batch.

> *Well, I guess it is time to admit that these small upticks in my weight really do bother me.*

Hey, that worked. I completely ignored my weight while I wrote those last few sentences. Hooray!

Day: #*31*   Weight: *192.*^6

Food & Water

7:00 a.m.	cappuccino		5:00 p.m.	peanut butter bar
7:30 a.m.	pills (1st B-12)		7:45 p.m.	chicken, cauliflower, broccoli
10:00 a.m.	cinnamon crunch bar			
11:00 a.m.	1st water done		8:30 p.m.	3rd water done
2:30 p.m.	sloppy joe		9:30 p.m.	maple, brown sugar oatmeal
2:45 p.m.	pill (2nd B-12)			
4:45 p.m.	2nd water done			

Exercise

None today.

Comments

According to my scale, this is the second day of an upward tick in my weight. Yikes! That is frustrating.

I guess, then, this is a mental test as much as anything else. I am not proud of how I am handling this area just yet.

I have got to concentrate and bear down.

I guess, then, this is a mental test as much as anything else.

48

Day: #*32*   Weight: *190.⁴*

Food & Water

7:15 a.m.	cappuccino
8:00 a.m.	pills (1st B-12)
10:15 a.m.	cinnamon crunch bar
10:30 a.m.	1st water done
1:15 p.m.	sloppy joe
1:30 p.m.	2nd water done
1:45 p.m.	pill (2nd B-12)

4:15 p.m.	peanut butter bar
7:00 p.m.	3rd water done
8:00 p.m.	talapia, cauliflower
10:00 p.m.	maple, brown sugar oatmeal
10:30 p.m.	4th water done

Exercise

Run: 15 minutes.
Weights: bench press (3 sets)

curls (bar) 3 sets
curls dumbbells (3 sets)

Comments

I hope this is the last note regarding the seesawing of my scale readings. This morning's numbers were down two whole pounds from yesterday.

Of course, it was just a correction from the two previous days when my weight climbed upward.

So, again, it balances out. Heretofore, however, I have been unable to ignore the erratic, wobbling trend.

In this instance, it works in my favor because it was a hefty drop. But, I must dismiss it and charge ahead.

My workout was excellent today. Interestingly, it only took a couple of sessions to get me back in the habit. I warmed up quickly and had plenty of vigor on each weight-lifting set.

I also noticed that I was a bit stronger. The weights moved slightly more easily.

I call it good progress.

49

Day: *#33*   Weight: *189.*[6]

Food & Water

8:15 a.m.	cappuccino	8:30 p.m.	turkey, zucchini
11:00 a.m.	cinnamon crunch bar	9:30 p.m.	pills (1st B-12)
1:00 p.m.	1st water done	10:00 p.m.	brownie
2:00 p.m.	sloppy joe	10:30 p.m.	pill (2nd B-12)
4:00 p.m.	2nd water done		
5:15 p.m.	peanut butter bar		
8:00 p.m.	3rd water done		

Exercise

None today.

Comments

When I consider how much exercise it takes to burn off those empty calories, it will be easy to resist those temptations.

Last night was Halloween. My wonderful children graciously offered to share their candy with me. Of course, I refused.

My boy was persistent. I had to insist that I had no interest and repeated offerings would be useless.

I never was a candy hog. But I certainly enjoyed a chocolate bar every few hours or so.

Now, however, I will be giving such treats many thoughts before indulging.

When I consider how much exercise it takes to burn off those empty calories, it will be easy to resist those temptations.

Day: #*34*   Weight: *189.²*

Food & Water

7:45 a.m.	cappuccino		7:30 p.m.	cod, broccoli, cauliflower
8:30 a.m.	pills (1st B-12)		9:15 p.m.	pill (2nd B-12)
10:00 a.m.	cinnamon crunch bar		9:30 p.m.	maple, brown sugar oatmeal
12:15 p.m.	1st water done		10:00 p.m.	3rd water done
12:45 p.m.	sloppy joe			
3:30 p.m.	peanut butter bar			
5:30 p.m.	2nd water done			

Exercise

None today.

Comments

My thoughts wandered a bit today. I remembered a previous time in my life when I lost a lot of weight.

I was very proud and quite happy with my size at the end of my weight-loss effort.

What I know now, however, has changed my opinion about the results I achieved. I was still technically overweight. I should have lost more.

Although I had done well, it was insufficient. I will be going all the way this time.

When it is all done, I will be unrecognizable to anyone who has known me over the previous few decades.

I will achieve a weight I have not experienced since I was in my teens. Look out world.

> *I will achieve a weight I have not experienced since I was in my teens. Look out world.*

Day: #*35* Weight: *188.*⁶

Food & Water

7:30 a.m.	cappuccino
9:45 a.m.	pills (1st B-12)
10:20 a.m.	cinnamon crunch bar
10:45 a.m.	1st water done
1:15 p.m.	sloppy joe
1:45 p.m.	second water done
4:15 p.m.	peanut butter bar
6:45 p.m.	3rd water done
7:15 p.m.	ground chicken, broccoli
8:30 p.m.	pill (2nd B-12)
10:45 p.m.	maple, brown sugar oatmeal

Exercise

Run: 15 minutes (alone)
Run: 15 minutes (with dog)

Weights: bench press (3 sets), curls (bar) (3 sets).

Comments

I had to go through my closet this morning to find dress slacks that don't sag on me like a parachute.

Turns out I even have to purchase a new pair of jeans.

I previously possessed a pile of pants representing a variety of sizes. I hope the need for such selection never arises again.

I hope my education and new habits developed from this program result in one set (size) of clothes and I can wear them until they fall off or go out of style.

A fit body, fortunately, will remain in vogue.

I previously possessed a pile of pants representing a variety of sizes. I hope the need for such selection never arises again.

AFTER FIVE WEEKS

IMPRESSIONS & PROGRESS

I had to dress fancier for an event at work today and a coworker commented that it was quite obvious my weight has dropped.

She said my face has changed and so has my body shape. I thanked her for the kind words and remarked that I have plenty of work still ahead of me.

At the event for which I had clothed myself so particularly, I saw an old friend. He had been showing some progress in his long, solo fight against unwanted body fat, but he noted how my results had quickly surpassed his.

Charged up, I became interested in increasing my exercise intensity. I know my ability will increase as I trim down and lighten up. The most important element, however, is the first step. That requires nothing more than me launching into workout sessions more frequently.

I can make that happen merely by putting in some extra initiative.

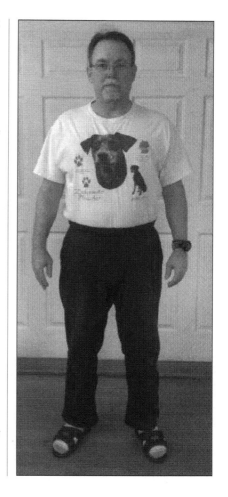

Day: #*36* Weight: *188.^{8}*

Food & Water

7:00 a.m.	cappuccino	4:00 p.m.	peanut butter bar
7:45 a.m.	pills (1st B-12)	4:10 p.m.	2nd water done
10:00 a.m.	cinnamon crunch bar	7:30 p.m.	ground chicken, broccoli
12:45 p.m.	1st water done	8:00 p.m.	3rd water done
1:15 p.m.	sloppy joe, ground turkey	10:00 p.m.	maple, brown sugar oatmeal
3:45 p.m.	pill (2nd B-12)		

Exercise

Swim: 20 laps, 30 minutes.

Comments

I went to the employee lounge to fill my bottle with ice this morning and the solitude afforded me a moment of thought.

It seems clear to me that most of my coworkers have not noticed I am getting lighter/smaller.

This can be attributed to my slow, gradual pace of weight loss.

For health reasons, a speedier drop is undesirable. I also need to note to myself that it is unimportant whether anyone recognizes my progress.

I am reminded daily of my continued success as my clothes keep getting baggier. My face keeps getting thinner. And my

For health reasons, a speedier drop is undesirable.

scale needle keeps heading south.

I get a daily reminder of my advancement via the full-length mirrors in my workplace elevators.

I also see my smile in there these days.

Day: #37   Weight: 189.⁰

Food & Water

7:15 a.m.	cappuccino
8:15 a.m.	pills (1st B-12)
9:45 a.m.	cinnamon crunch bar
11:00 a.m.	1st water done
12:45 p.m.	sloppy joe, turkey
1:15 p.m.	pill (2nd B-12)
1:30 p.m.	2nd water done

4:00 p.m.	peanut butter bar
7:15 p.m.	talapia, zucchini
10:00 p.m.	chocolate pudding
10:15 p.m.	3rd water done

Exercise

None today.

Comments

At work, there was a board meeting scheduled, so I was fully accessorized with a coat and tie.

This is only relevant because dress clothes are a considerable pain to negotiate when I go to the pool at lunch.

So, this burden was on my mind when I had to decide whether to swim laps today.

The clothing issue made me alter my favorite plan and tell myself I would instead run the neighborhood after work.

Of course, when the time to get fleeting feet arrived, I was busy with kids' homework and other routine tasks at the house.

Procrastination is an adversary that bears watching closely.

And that is how the day ended without a check in the exercise column.

Procrastination is an adversary that bears watching closely.

Day: #*38*   Weight: *189.*[6]

Food & Water

7:00 a.m.	cappuccino
10:00 a.m.	cinnamon crunch bar
12:30 p.m.	1st water done
12:45 p.m.	pills (1st B-12)
1:00 p.m.	sloppy joe
4:00 p.m.	peanut butter bar
5:00 p.m.	pill (2nd B-12)

5:30 p.m.	2nd water done
7:00 p.m.	ground chicken, turkey, broccoli
9:30 p.m.	maple, brown sugar oatmeal
10:00 p.m.	3rd water done

Exercise

Swim: 20 laps, 25 minutes.

Comments

This morning as I was getting dressed it dawned on me again how much more easily I can maneuver my body now that a significant amount of fat is gone.

It may seem humorous to some people, but in previous days, it was uncomfortable just putting on a pair of socks.

Now I have an easier time reaching my feet and moving them into position for the task at hand.

I hope I don't take such flexibility for granted in the future. I hope I continue to appreciate it always as much as I do right now.

I saw my reflection in a large window as I got out of the pool after my swim. It confirmed two things: 1) I am not a vampire as some folks may have believed and 2) I still have a long way to go.

I won't let that horrible image discourage me, but someone should throw a big blanket up to cover that glass—or at least to cover me.

Day: #*39*   Weight: *188.²*

Food & Water

7:00 a.m.	cappuccino
10:00 a.m.	cinnamon crunch bar
10:05 a.m.	pills (1st B-12)
1:00 p.m.	sloppy joe, turkey
2:15 p.m.	pill (2nd B-12)
2:30 p.m.	1st water done
4:00 p.m.	peanut butter bar

5:30 p.m.	2nd water done
7:30 p.m.	cod, broccoli
10:00 p.m.	3rd water done
10:30 p.m.	chocolate pudding

Exercise

None today.

Comments

My thoughts today don't seem directly related to my diet. But I wonder if they are related indirectly and significantly.

What I mean is, my work environment put me into a gloomy mood. I spent some time contemplating how much my mental attitude could affect my body's efforts to burn calories.

I could be wrong, but I like to think a good mood and attitude have a distinctly positive effect on us physically.

Wouldn't the opposite, then, also be true?

I am puzzled. I suppose there is no real way to know for sure.

I could be wrong, but I like to think a good mood and attitude have a distinctly positive effect on us physically.

Day: #*40*   Weight: *186.*^{8}

Food & Water

8:30 a.m.	cappuccino		4:30 p.m.	3rd water done
9:30 a.m.	pills (1st B-12)		5:00 p.m.	peanut butter bar
11:30 a.m.	cinnamon crunch bar		8:30 p.m.	ground chickem, broccoli
12:00 p.m.	1st water done		10:30 p.m.	brownie
2:30 p.m.	2nd water done		10:45 p.m.	4th water done
3:00 p.m.	sloppy joe			
5:00 p.m.	pill (2nd B-12)			

Exercise

None today.

Comments

I really, really wanted to exercise today. I knew I would have trouble getting it done because I am charged with looking after my kids all day.

Still, I thought I at least would be able to hit the garage for a few minutes to tackle my weight bench. I could have checked on the kids between sets.

I figured that, if I were exceptionally lucky, I could get their older sister to keep an eye on them for about 15 or 20 minutes while I ran.

Absolutely no luck came my way.

So, the day is ending as I write

Absolutely no luck came my way.

this. It is too late for a strenuous physical workout. I must take all the precautions to ensure there are no obstacles interfering with my schedule tomorrow. I know; these are the realities of adult life and we must do our best and keep trying.

Day: #*41*   Weight: *186.*⁴

Food & Water

7:45 a.m.	cappuccino		5:00 p.m.	3rd water done
9:45 a.m.	pills (1st B-12)		5:30 p.m.	sloppy joe
11:15 a.m.	cinnamon crunch bar		8:00 p.m.	ground pork, broccoli
12:00 p.m.	1st water done		8:45 p.m.	4th water done
1:15 p.m.	2nd water done		10:15 p.m.	brownie
1:45 p.m.	pill (2nd B-12)			
2:15 p.m.	peanut butter bar			

Exercise

Run: 30 minutes (15 with kids) (15 with dog). Weights: bench, 3 sets; curls (bar), 3 sets; curls (dumbbells) 3 sets.

Comments

Today was incredible. I had a good opportunity to exercise because it was Sunday. I took advantage of it.

Unfortunately, I overdid it. I went for a run and the kids came along. That is always special.

When we got back, the wife wanted me to take the dog for a jog, too. Off I went.

When the running was through, I was warmed up and feeling like hitting the weights was a good idea. It was.

After that, I was feeling "productive" so I finished painting the trim on our house. It was tough on my arms, since I had to use an extended pole.

Next I climbed the hill out front to lop the thick-trunked weeds that were spreading and rising too high.

By the time I neared the end of clipping them for the bins, my arms were giving out. I was spent.

It is after 9 p.m. as I write this note and I am still exhausted. I still have to eat again in an hour. So, I am unable to lie down to sleep yet.

Day: #*42*   Weight: *186.*⁸

Food & Water

7:00 a.m.	cappuccino
9:45 a.m.	pills (1st B-12)
10:00 a.m.	cinnamon crunch bar
10:15 a.m.	1st water done
1:00 p.m.	sloppy joe
1:15 p.m.	2nd water done
1:30 p.m.	pill (2nd B-12)

4:00 p.m.	peanut butter bar
7:15 p.m.	ground chickem, zucchini
7:30 p.m.	3rd water done
10:30 p.m.	maple, brown sugar oatmeal

Exercise

Run: 15 minutes (with dog).

Comments

After yesterday's brutal bout with exercise and yard work, I was afraid I would be unable to move my limbs today.

Fortunately, seven hours of sleep washed away the exhaustion. I was left with only sore muscles.

I don't mind that. In fact, I think of it as a reminder that my weight lifting is having a positive effect.

My run was pretty routine. I stretched out fairly well so pain in my legs and feet was minimal.

As each foot pounded the roadway, it made me remember that my body is still way too heavy. I have lost about a third of what I plan to lose in this program.

I've got work to do.

> *As each foot pounded the roadway, it made me remember that my body is still way too heavy.*

AFTER SIX WEEKS

IMPRESSIONS & PROGRESS

Wow! A lousy two pounds is all I've lost this week.

I know it is supposed to average out to be between that and three pounds per week, but this slowing trend is really bothering me.

I am working hard and eating exactly what I am supposed to without even the slightest variation. I want to see better results, bigger losses.

Worse than shedding only a pittance this week is the fact that I am in a several-day slump. I certainly am experiencing a dreaded plateau.

I suppose I should try to stay positive, even in these tough times. My total so far is just over 20 pounds.

It is excellent to be 20 pounds lighter. It is only diminished when I remember that it is but one-third of the total weight I need to drop.

Oops, there I go again....

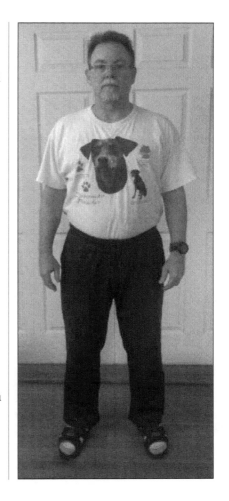

Day: #*43*   Weight: *186.*[6]

Food & Water

8:00 a.m.   cappuccino
9:00 a.m.   pills (1st B-12)
11:00 a.m. cinnamon crunch bar
11:05 a.m. 1st water done
2:15 p.m.   beef vegetable soup
5:15 p.m.   peanut butter bar
6:45 p.m.   2nd water done

7:00 p.m.   pill (2nd B-12)
8:00 p.m.   ground chickem,
            turkey, broccoli
8:30 p.m.   3rd water done
9:30 p.m.   chocolate pudding

Exercise

None today.

Comments

Today was significant. For the first time in my participation in this diet program, I am giving serious consideration to parting ways with my counselor and continuing on as a solo act.

I am doubting the value of my weekly visits. According to established plan, I was supposed to "grope the robot" today.

I look forward to the machine's detailed analysis. It allows me to know whether I am burning or building muscle. Since I rarely have any questions, and the only remaining activity is to take my blood pressure (occasionally), my visits may have minimal importance.

...I am giving serious consideration to parting ways with my counselor...

I can check my own blood pressure, although it probably is unnecessary, and I can buy the food on the Internet. Therefore, I must give this some deliberation.

Day: #*44*   Weight: *186.⁶*

Food & Water

7:00 a.m.	cappuccino
8:00 a.m.	pills (1st B-12)
10:00 a.m.	cinnamon crunch bar
12:15 p.m.	1st water done
1:15 p.m.	beef vegetable soup
1:45 p.m.	pill (2nd B-12)
4:10 p.m.	2nd water done

4:20 p.m.	peanut butter bar
6:30 p.m.	3rd water done
7:30 p.m.	ground chicken, turkey, zucchini
10:15 p.m.	chocolate pudding
10:40 p.m.	4th water done

Exercise

None today.

Comments

My weight today is exactly the same as it was yesterday. For the last few days, I have been trapped in a small window of scale readings.

I am not fretting, however. I am thus anticipating a significant drop any day now because there is no legitimate reason for a halt to my weight-loss trend.

It had better "bust a move" pretty soon, though.

Since I forgot my book for my last meeting with my counselor, I scanned the pages and emailed them to her.

Seeing the entries side-by-side, I noticed that my weight actually has been in the same whole number for five consecutive days.

Yes, this blockage had better jettison itself quick-like or there will be trouble.

...there is no legitimate reason for a halt to my weight-loss trend.

Day: #*45* Weight: *187.⁰*

Food & Water

7:00 a.m.   cappuccino
9:00 a.m.   pills (1st B-12)
10:15 a.m. cinnamon crunch bar
11:45 a.m. 1st water done
1:30 p.m.   sloppy joe
2:10 p.m.   pill (2nd B-12)
4:15 p.m.   peanut butter bar

7:30 p.m.   ground pork, broccoli
9:00 p.m.   3rd water done
10:30 p.m. brownie

Exercise

None today.

Comments

Okay, serious frustration is hitting me today. This is my seventh day in a row with no weight loss.

In fact, it has risen slightly after having hovered for the previous six days.

They said there will be plateaus. I had prepared myself after experiencing smaller but similar setbacks.

But a full week without progress is making me have significant doubts. I am not truly considering quitting just yet. But I am going to be more critical.

If my weight doesn't begin trending downward soon, I will be asking the good folks who monitor me to explain why I should continue with their program.

If their answer fails to impress, I may have to branch out and use my own program that has been successful in the past.

This is my seventh day in a row with no weight loss.

Day: #*46*   Weight: *185.⁶*

Food & Water

7:00 a.m.	cappuccino
8:30 a.m.	pills (1st B-12)
10:00 a.m.	cinnamon crunch bar
12:25 p.m.	1st water done
1:00 p.m.	peanut butter bar
3:45 p.m.	pill (2nd B-12)
4:00 p.m.	2nd water done
4:15 p.m.	sloppy joe
7:00 p.m.	3rd water done
8:30 p.m.	ground chicken, broccoli
10:30 p.m.	chocolate shake

Exercise

Weights: bench press, 3 sets; curls (bar) 3 sets, curls (dumbbells) 3 sets. Run: 15 minutes (with dog).

Comments

Donuts in the lounge! I just shook my head and felt thankful to work in a place with people who are so willing to share goodies.

Passing on the delectables might not have been so easy had my scale not finally shown a downward move this morning.

Yes, after a full week of stagnation, the needle (digital readout) showed a pound-and-a-half drop.

I would get excited, but it just as easily could rise tomorrow. So, head down and lean forward, I say.

It is not a sprint but a long march to the finish line—which remains near the horizon.

Donuts in the lounge! ...Passing on the delectables might not have been so easy had my scale not finally shown a downward move this morning.

Day: #**47**   Weight: **185.**⁶

Food & Water

8:45 a.m.	cappuccino
9:45 a.m.	pills (1st B-12)
11:30 a.m.	1st water done
11:45 a.m.	cinnamon crunch bar
3:00 p.m.	beef vegetable soup
3:30 p.m.	2nd water done
5:30 p.m.	pill (2nd B-12)
6:00 p.m.	peanut butter bar
6:15 p.m.	3rd water done
8:00 p.m.	ground chicken, turkey, broccoli
10:30 p.m.	chocolate shake

Exercise

None today.

Comments

Ignoring the scale readings and pressing on is the only acceptable response to these 'slowdowns.'

I awoke this morning to the exact same weight I was yesterday.

I am not upset, though. If it turns out to be another string of days with no movement, then I will give serious consideration to getting angry.

Not that there is anything I really can do about it. Ignoring the scale readings and pressing on is the only acceptable response to these "slowdowns."

Day: #48   Weight: 185.⁶

Food & Water

8:00 a.m.	cappuccino
9:15 a.m.	pills (1st B-12)
11:00 a.m.	cinnamon crunch bar
11:45 a.m.	1st water done
1:45 p.m.	peanut butter bar
4:30 p.m.	2nd water done
5:15 p.m.	beef vegetable soup
7:30 p.m.	ground chicken, turkey, broccoli
10:00 p.m.	3rd water done
10:05 p.m.	pill (2nd B-12)
10:15 p.m.	maple, brown sugar oatmeal

Exercise

Run: 15 minutes (with dog); Weights: Squats, 3 sets; military press, 3 sets.

Comments

My morning weigh-in is getting to be like the movie, "Groundhog Day."

Today is the third day of the exact same scale reading. The previous number went for seven days.

Is this the new normal? Will I go from plateau to plateau? It shouldn't matter, I suppose, as long as the overall trend is downward.

I know this in my head, but it causes me some deliberation every time it actually happens.

My run was good. My weight-lifting routine was mixed to enjoy some variety.

The military press worked some muscles I have been neglecting. It was good to stress them again. I need to get them into the schedule more frequently.

I worked my legs, too, in a way that running is unable to do. Jogging helps build endurance, but squats build muscle mass, increasing their size and calorie-burning capacity.

Day: #*49*   Weight: *185.*⁸

Day: #*49*   Weight: $185.^{8}$

Food & Water

7:30 a.m.	cappuccino
7:45 a.m.	pills (1st B-12)
10:30 a.m.	cinnamon crunch bar
12:00 p.m.	1st water done
1:30 p.m.	peanut butter bar
4:30 p.m.	pill (2nd B-12)
4:45 p.m.	2nd water done

5:00 p.m.	sloppy joe
7:30 p.m.	ground chicken, turkey, broccoli
10:00 p.m.	maple, brown sugar oatmeal
10:05 p.m.	3rd water done

Exercise

None today.

Comments

I hate to dwell on the topic, but this is my fourth day of the same weight.

I have an appointment with my program counselor in the morning and I am quite concerned that I will have nearly no weight loss to show for my efforts.

I have had a series of flat spells and this recent one is still upon me. I will be lucky to see a one-pound dip at tomorrow's weigh-in.

One good thing: I should get to "grope the robot" and see a breakdown of my body composition.

I am hoping it tells me that I

I will be lucky to see a one-pound dip...

have been gaining muscle and that is why my weight is dropping so slowly.

If that is the case, it will be okay because it will mean my body is getting into better shape.

Knowing that, I can better deal with this snail's pace.

Total pounds lost so far:
21.²

AFTER SEVEN WEEKS

IMPRESSIONS & PROGRESS

It was a rough week. At least a few times I felt like quitting. I even threatened such an action in my thoughts.

It was all the result of serious frustration. My weight leveled out and stayed almost motionless for a week.

I had been warned such plateaus would sneak into my program. I thought I was ready for them.

They are a different matter when they actually materialize. That can be seen easily by reading my daily notes. I thought I was going to burst.

In the end (of the week, at least), however, there was little chance of me giving up now. I will ride it out indefinitely because I am seeing good results overall.

Daily disturbances ("frozen" scale readings) must be tolerated. I can and will refocus and bear down.

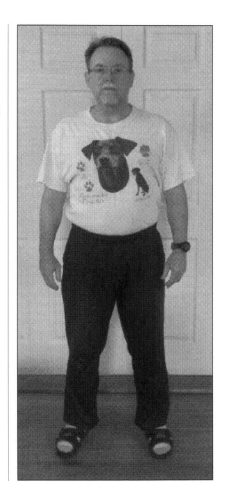

Day: #*50*   Weight: *185.*[4]

Food & Water

7:00 a.m.	cappuccino
7:45 a.m.	pills (1st B-12)
10:00 a.m.	cinnamon crunch bar
12:00 p.m.	1st water done
1:00 p.m.	sloppy joe
3:00 p.m.	2nd water done
4:45 p.m.	peanut butter bar

5:00 p.m.	3rd water done
7:30 p.m.	ground chicken, broccoli
8:00 p.m.	pill (2nd B-12)
10:00 p.m.	peanut butter soft serve

Exercise

None today.

Comments

Apparently, however, the new norm is for scale readings to stagnate for a few days and then plop a pound or so.

Well, my date with the computer confirmed that I am still dropping weight, overall.

Apparently, however, the new norm is for scale readings to stagnate for a few days and then plop a pound or so.

I have no choice but to accept this new way of shrinking. Fighting it will be of no use.

Resistance, as they say, is futile.

Day: #*51*   Weight: *184.*⁴

Food & Water

7:00 a.m.   cappuccino
7:20 a.m.   pills (1st B-12)
10:00 a.m. cinnamon crunch bar
10:20 a.m. 1st water done
12:45 p.m. maple, brown sugar
           oatmeal
3:45 p.m.   peanut butter bar

4:15 p.m.   pill (2nd B-12)
6:00 p.m.   2nd water done
7:15 p.m.   talapia, zucchini
10:00 p.m. peanut butter soft
           serve
10:30 p.m. 3rd water done

Exercise

None today.

Comments

Now it is time to focus on increasing exercise to efficiently burn more calories and build more muscle to increase my body's minimum at-rest calorie usage.

So, today's weigh-in revealed a full one-pound drop from yesterday. That seems to confirm the new pattern.

I will be rolling steady at the weigh-ins until—blam!—the scale shows a plunge.

So be it.

Now it is time to focus on increasing exercise to efficiently burn more calories and build more muscle to increase my body's minimum at-rest calorie usage.

All that will create better balance, better health, better weight, better attitude (mental tranquility).

Day: #*52*   Weight: *183.*⁸

Food & Water

7:15 a.m.	cappuccino	4:20 p.m.	2nd water done
9:00 a.m.	pills (1st B-12)	7:30 p.m.	ground chicken, cauliflower, broccoli
10:30 a.m.	cinnamon crunch bar	8:30 p.m.	3rd water done
12:45 p.m.	1st water done	10:00 p.m.	peanut butter soft serve
1:15 p.m.	maple, brown sugar oatmeal	10:30 p.m.	pill (2nd B-12)
4:15 p.m.	peanut butter bar		

Exercise

None today.

Comments

Second day in a row with registered weight loss. Has the pattern officially changed?

I hope this is a trend.

I talked myself out of swimming today. I set my sights on a good run of the neighborhood with my faithful pooch, Abby.

Then I got news I would be working late again. See how things happen?

It is the curse of procrastination. Putting off for later so often seems to backfire. Logical plans routinely get crushed.

I better work on the follow-through some more. Oh, and the muscles, too.

Putting off for later so often seems to backfire. Logical plans routinely get crushed.

Day: #*53*   Weight: *183.*⁶

Food & Water

7:00 a.m.	cappuccino
9:30 a.m.	pills (1st B-12)
10:45 a.m.	cinnamon crunch bar
1:15 p.m.	1st water done
1:45 p.m.	sloppy joe
4:30 p.m.	pill (2nd B-12)
4:45 p.m.	peanut butter bar

5:10 p.m.	2nd water done
7:45 p.m.	chicken, broccoli
10:30 p.m.	peanut butter soft serve
11:00 p.m.	3rd water done

Exercise

None today.

Comments

Another small drop in weight. That's a good thing. Maybe I am returning to a "slow and steady" pattern.

I withstood... uh... enjoyed my own birthday last night. Previous habits were to feast heavily at a local restaurant.

That failed to fit well into this diet program. So the family stayed home.

My holiday meal was ground chicken, cauliflower and broccoli. It was awesome and I couldn't be happier. My kids and wife made great cards for me and gave me nice presents.

What an excellent day. And I woke up lighter, too! Can't beat that.

> *My holiday meal was ground chicken, cauliflower and broccoli. It was awesome and I couldn't be happier.*

73

Day: **#54**   Weight: **183.**[6]

Food & Water

7:30 a.m.	cappuccino		7:15 p.m.	3rd water done
9:15 a.m.	pills (1st B-12)		8:30 p.m.	ground pork,
10:30 a.m.	cinnamon crunch bar			cauliflower, broccoli
11:45 a.m.	1st water done		9:00 p.m.	pill (2nd B-12)
1:30 p.m.	peanut butter bar		10:15 p.m.	peanut butter soft
3:30 p.m.	2nd water done			serve
5:00 p.m.	beef & vegetable soup			

Exercise

None today.

Comments

Today can be described as mediocre.

I mean there is absolutely nothing special about it. My morning leap onto the scale showed my weight hasn't changed beyond yesterday's number.

But this is not notable. I am getting used to those flattenings. So, I was neither excited nor gloomy as I carried out the day's routine.

I cannot complain. All that means is that the day would be whatever I made it.

That's a pretty good deal. And I think I did it justice.

I took the kids out so they

I cannot complain. ...the day would be whatever I made it.

could have lunch and play to burn some energy.

We also did some browsing in a hat store. They began to get wild among the displays, so we left.

Tomorrow is a new start.

Day: #*55*   Weight: *182.*⁴

Food & Water

8:30 a.m.	cappuccino
9:30 a.m.	pills (1st B-12)
11:40 a.m.	cinnamon crunch bar
12:50 p.m.	1st water done
3:15 p.m.	sloppy joe
3:30 p.m.	2nd water done
6:00 p.m.	3rd water done
6:15 p.m.	peanut butter bar
8:30 p.m.	cod, broccoli
8:45 p.m.	pill (2nd B-12)
10:30 p.m.	chocolate shake
10:40 p.m.	4th water done

Exercise

Run: 15 minutes (with dog).
Weights: bench press, 3 sets; military press, 3 sets.

Comments

I don't work today, but my canine pal insisted I let her out at 6:30 a.m.

That is her usual, weekday time and she is clueless about my days off and holidays.

I felt no aggravation. I got up and began my routine.

The scale delighted me with a favorable reading. I am more than a pound lower than yesterday.

I bounced to the kitchen to mix and heat my cappuccino.

That put me in a good mood, too, so I made the wife's coffee.

The gang went to a birthday party, so I had some time to hit the stores for a new pair of jeans.

The pair I have been wearing has gotten uncomfortably large. I know they are but a couple of weeks old, but my waist is shrinking.

I am not complaining about the cost of clothing renewal.

66

The scale delighted me...

99

Day: #*56*   Weight: *182.*⁴

Food & Water

7:15 a.m.	cappuccino		7:15 p.m.	2nd water done
7:45 a.m.	pills (1st B-12)		7:45 p.m.	pork chop, broccoli
10:15 a.m.	cinnamon crunch bar		10:30 p.m.	3rd water done
10:55 a.m.	1st water done		10:45 p.m.	chocolate shake
1:30 p.m.	sloppy joe			
1:35 p.m.	pill (2nd B-12)			
4:30 p.m.	peanut butter bar			

Exercise

None today.

Comments

Ah, another day and no weight change. I didn't give it another thought all day, however.

I did have several episodes of visions of a new me. That reality is a long way off, though.

I haven't even reached the halfway point yet. That's an odd situation. I feel like I have dropped plenty of weight and my body has changed its shape and appearance.

But I only have reached the status of "fairly overweight person" instead of the ridiculously obese slob I was several weeks ago.

That is not a magnificant accomplishment.

I want to be happy about my achievement, but it is so small.

I guess I am just a bit gloomy today overall and I am focusing on my weight and putting the blame there.

I must do better at this mental game of dieting.

The mind is too big an element to ignore or even take lightly.

AFTER EIGHT WEEKS

IMPRESSIONS & PROGRESS

Well, my weight-loss pattern remains jagged. That is not news, though.

I must remind myself, however, about procrastination. I was guilty of that recently. I put off a lunch-time swim, intending to run instead that night. I had to work late.

One of last week's days was the anniversary of my birth. The family skipped the usual restaurant feast and got together at our house. I am unable to remember what everyone else ate, but my dinner was ground chicken and vegetables. I loved it. We got cake for the kids. No need for them to miss that fun. They blew out a few candles for me, too.

My total weight loss so far is about 25 pounds. That is good, but I am not halfway to my goal yet. Still, I can't complain. I did purchase a new pair of jeans the other day because the previous pair, bought a couple of weeks earlier, became uncomfortably baggy.

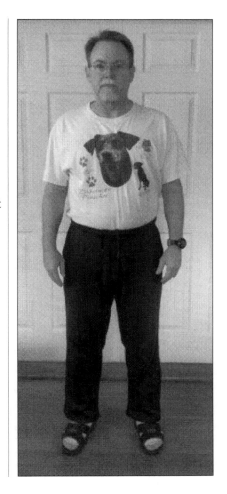

4

Trimmed to visual proof, learning still

The second month of my participation in this diet program was marked by significant and visible weight loss.

I am not just referring to watching the scale readings drop. I am talking about notable alterations to my body.

For example, I had to adjust my watchband. Big deal, you say? Okay, I also have a favorite hat that I have been unable to wear for a couple of years because it was too tight.

It now fits quite comfortably.

I also have dealt with the obvious changes. I have had to purchase new pants and belts.

And, I am wearing smaller jackets (blazers) and sweatshirts that previously were impossible to don without looking like a squeezed turnip.

The last part of this visible shift pertains to my legs. I had not realized how puffy they were until I saw them at their current, shrunken state.

Believe me; it is quite a good feeling to see your own stilts all trimmed down.

It made me say to myself, "Never again will I let that happen."

I mean that it is one thing to get a little flabby around the gut. It is something entirely different to pack on so many additional pounds that they spread themselves from your head to your toes. No more, I say.

The period also was a time

when I became even more enthused about exercise. I am sure I never will evolve into one of those people who live and breathe for aerobics or weight lifting.

You know the type. They end up making videos to sell to fat-loss followers.

But I do see myself working some physical activities into my weekly routine, enough to keep me in shape for life.

I have no doubts about accomplishing this goal, since exercise keeps getting easier and more enjoyable as my body continues to get lighter and better shaped.

So, look for me out on the road. I will be running or bicycling or some other form of workout that is even more interesting and beneficial.

And this diet so far has taught me that it will not take much to maintain proper weight once I get there.

It will be far simpler to keep off the excess fat than to burn it away in the first place.

There also were points in the past month that were not at all pleasant.

I had to come to grips with the knowledge that I would only be losing about two pounds per week.

I know I had been told this,

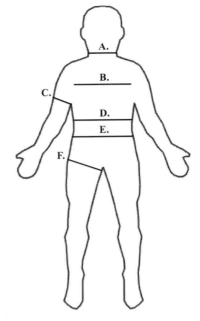

A. Neck: 16

B. Chest: 44

C. Biceps: 13

D. Waist (navel): $39.^5$

E. High Hip (belt line): 37

F. Thighs: 23

G. Weight: $182.^4$

but I felt like I could burn it faster. And I probably can, but that would be an unhealthy speed.

Suffice it to say I was a bit frustrated by the finality of that pace.

But, I eventually settled down and accepted it.

What really angered me, however, were a few flat spots in my weight decline.

My weight-loss pattern was odd. It would bounce up and down for days, staying very close to a particular whole number before finally dropping and letting me know we were back in business.

This routine proved to be difficult, even though I had been warned about it.

I even thought about quitting the program. I thought that more than once.

Fortunately, I came to my senses before I did anything dumb. I have learned to accept those plateaus as well.

So, I suppose the best way to describe the second month of my diet program is as a learning experience.

I had thought the first month exposed me to everything, at least enough for me to feel like I was a pro. I guess this diet still has a few surprises for this old dog.

I must remain open to learning some new tricks.

Day: #*57*   Weight: *181.*⁶

Food & Water

7:15 a.m.	cappuccino
8:10 a.m.	pills (1st B-12)
10:30 a.m.	cinnamon crunch bar
11:20 a.m.	1st water done
12:30 p.m.	salmon, broccoli
3:30 p.m.	peanut butter bar
5:00 p.m.	pill (2nd B-12)

6:10 p.m.	2nd water done
7:05 p.m.	peanut butter bar
9:15 p.m.	3rd water done
9:30 p.m.	chocolate pudding

Exercise

None today.

Comments

The program allows moving any of the meals to any time of the day.

Today was the first time I changed up my eating schedule.

I had my "normal" meal at lunchtime. Normally that is my dinner, which I enjoy while sitting and talking with my family.

It is perfectly acceptable to make such an alteration. The program allows moving any of the meals to any time of the day.

That is no issue. It is only a matter of how I will handle dinner time with a peanut butter bar or some similar snack-size meal. I will not know for another couple of hours.

Update: I got through it. But I prefer my regular schedule.

Day: #*58*   Weight: *180.⁶*

Food & Water

7:00 a.m.	cappuccino
7:45 a.m.	pills (1st B-12)
10:15 a.m.	lemon meringue bar
1:00 p.m.	maple, brown sugar oatmeal
1:15 p.m.	1st water done
4:15 p.m.	chocolate bar

4:45 p.m.	pill (2nd B-12)
5:15 p.m.	2nd water done
8:00 p.m.	ground chicken, broccoli
10:30 p.m.	chocolate pudding
10:35 p.m.	3rd water done

Exercise

None today.

Comments

Will I ever eat another donut? I am sure I will, but I will be in a better place mentally...

Donuts in the lounge again.

This is so commonplace that I am unable to use an exclamation mark to end that sentence.

They had several of my most favorite kinds. Happily, I walked on by.

Will I ever eat another donut? I'm sure I will, but I will be in a better place mentally and will be sure to offset it with reduced eating at other times and vigorous exercise.

Donuts and junk food are not enemies. They are temptations that can be controlled. I am winning that battle.

83

Day: #*59*   Weight: *181.*²

Food & Water

8:15 a.m.	cappuccino		7:00 p.m.	ground chicken, broccoli
9:45 a.m.	pills (1st B-12)			
11:30 a.m.	lemon meringue bar		7:05 p.m.	mashed potatoes
12:45 p.m.	1st water done		7:30 p.m.	3rd water done
2:30 p.m.	mashed potatoes		9:30 p.m.	chocolate pudding
3:00 p.m.	pill (2nd B-12)			
3:30 p.m.	2nd water done			

Exercise

Run: 15 minutes (w/son & dog); Weights: bench press, 3 sets; military press, 3 sets; curls (bar) 3 sets.

Comments

It is Thanksgiving Day.

Leading up to this, people who know I am dieting asked how I would handle the holiday meal. Would I take a day off and devour massive amounts of food?

My response was the same to each of them: I will stick to the program. I have no idea how badly my progress might be stalled by one day, one meal, or even one bite that fails to conform to the plan's specifications.

I really don't want any success I have already achieved to be wasted by a temporary enjoyment of some vittles.

Actually, with my current attitude, I doubt I would find an alternate meal very likable.

So I will be thankful that I have accomplished some weight loss so far, that my family is all together today, that we have a comfortable home and that we are all in good health.

Happy Thanksgiving to us.

Wait! Is that pumpkin pie I smell?

(Just kidding.)

Day: #*60*   Weight: *180.*⁴

Food & Water

8:00 a.m.	cappuccino		oatmeal
9:00 a.m.	pills (1st B-12)	8:00 p.m.	ground chicken,
11:30 a.m.	lemon meringue bar		broccoli
12:20 p.m.	1st water done	9:00 p.m.	3rd water done
2:30 p.m.	chocolate bar	9:45 p.m.	peanut butter soft
2:45 p.m.	2nd water done		serve
5:30 p.m.	apple cinnamon		

Exercise

Run: 15 minutes (w/dog).

Comments

I had a nice little drop in weight as told by the scale this morning.

It had risen slightly yesterday. But it probably only looks that way based on the reading from the day before.

That morning was a strange situation. I weighed myself when I first awoke in the a.m. That is my routine.

I weighed myself again, however, about 10 minutes later when I got out of the shower.

Oddly, the latter reading was lower. And that is the weight I recorded. Of course, the following day's setup was only one reading and it appeared in comparison to jump-up the result.

But, I believe all is back to normal.

I am only going to take one scale reading in the morning and that will be at the same time I have taken the previous 50 readings—before standing in the rain locker.

Day: #*61*   Weight: *180.*⁶

Food & Water

8:30 a.m.	cappuccino
9:45 a.m.	pills (1st B-12)
11:30 a.m.	lemon meringue bar
2:45 p.m.	apple cinnamon oatmeal
2:55 p.m.	1st water done
5:15 p.m.	chocolate bar
6:10 p.m.	2nd water done
7:05 p.m.	pill (2nd B-12)
9:00 p.m.	talapia, spinach
9:30 p.m.	3rd water done
10:30 p.m.	chocolate shake

Exercise

None today.

Comments

This morning's scale reading was up two-tenths of a pound.

It is no big deal. I guess I really am getting used to the hovering and slowdowns.

Since it has no effect on my attitude, I can pursue my daily routine without disappointment.

Since I had talapia—the leanest protein—tonight, I needed to add a good fat. I used a lite salad dressing on my spinach.

That "zesty" Italian taste was a nice treat. I guess I am forced to pair the leaves with fish because I cannot see eating that green stuff raw. That is, without something to "dress" it up for my taste buds.

Maybe I will try it naked (the vegetable) and see how my palate handles it.

Maybe I will try it naked (the vegetable) and see how my palate handles it.

Day: #*62* Weight: *180.*²

Food & Water

7:30 a.m.	cappuccino
9:45 a.m.	pills (1st B-12)
10:30 a.m.	lemon meringue bar
10:50 a.m.	1st water done
2:15 p.m.	apple cinnamon
	oatmeal
2:25 p.m.	2nd water done

5:00 p.m.	chocolate bar
8:00 p.m.	ground chicken,
	broccoli
8:15 p.m.	3rd water done
8:45 p.m.	pill (2nd B-12)
9:00 p.m.	chocolate pudding

Exercise

Run: 15 minutes (w/dog).
Weights: bench press, 3 sets; curls (bar) 3 sets; military press, 3 sets; squats, 3 sets.

Comments

My scale is a slow mover again. Fortunately, it is a downward angle.

It is Sunday. It could be a lazy one. I have plenty of ways to spend time on my computer, but the hours would be better spent if I got some exercise underway early.

A good morning workout will energize me and set a good tone for the rest of the day.

I just finished my run with the dog and that is getting easier. I mean that I am able to run faster and farther in the same amount of time. That demonstrates improvement.

Some comes from weight loss alone. The rest comes from regular running and an endurance buildup.

It is all going as planned.

I finally tried the cereal of the packaged-food lineup. It was my first and last time.

Chomping them dry was not going to be filling. Wetting them with water made them into something disgusting.

Day: #**63**   Weight: **180.**⁰

Food & Water

7:45 a.m.	cappuccino
8:00 a.m.	pills (1st B-12)
11:00 a.m.	lemon meringue bar
12:30 p.m.	1st water done
1:30 p.m.	chocolate bar
6:00 p.m.	2nd water done
6:20 p.m.	chocolate shake

7:30 p.m.	talapia, spinach
7:45 p.m.	3rd water done
8:00 p.m.	pill (2nd B-12)
8:30 p.m.	cereal

Exercise

None today.

Comments

I woke up this morning like it was any other day. It developed into something terrible, however.

As the day progressed, I felt more and more ill. I am not completely surprised. My wife was in similar shape the day before yesterday.

It is especially problematic for me because of my diet plan eating schedule. I am lost for how to accomplish it while I have zero appetite.

More than that, I am unable to imagine eating anything. My stomach is a bit pained. I almost feel I need to vomit.

I also am feeling cold and very weak. I just want to go to bed.

I'll try to force down the required food, but I am worried. I am wishing myself luck.

I found a way to move forward. I am "drinking" the remainder of my five meals.

I have to give some thought to handling the "normal" meal.

Did I mention the back pain?

88

AFTER NINE WEEKS

IMPRESSIONS & PROGRESS

Thanksgiving fell within my ninth week. Friends seemed concerned the holiday would spell disaster for me.

I love filling my pie hole with holiday goodies as much as anyone else.

I am on a mission, though, and I have the willpower to refrain from endeavoring in such counterproductive behavior.

I do not mean to set myself on a pedestal. My intention is to explain that I have changed my attitude toward meals.

I have adjusted my thinking to accept that meals are a way to sustain life and they should not be thought of as magical treats for the taste buds.

I still enjoy meals and I will enjoy them more again after I complete the program. But I will not get stupid at this point in time and take a chance at slowing my progress. I was thankful for health and family. Food played no part in that.

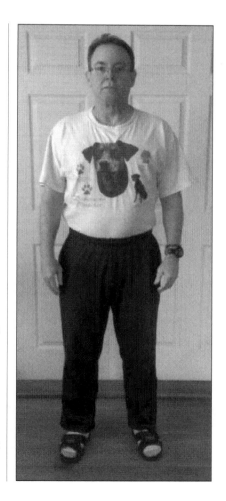

Day: #**64**   Weight: **180.**⁴

Food & Water

7:15 a.m.	cappuccino		7:00 p.m.	ground chicken, broccoli
7:45 a.m.	pills (1st B-12)			
10:15 a.m.	lemon meringue bar		8:30 p.m.	2nd water done
10:25 a.m.	1st water done		9:45 p.m.	pill (2nd B-12)
1:30 p.m.	chocolate shake		10:00 p.m.	cappuccino (decaf)
4:30 p.m.	chocolate bar		10:00 p.m.	3rd water done

Exercise

None today.

Comments

I wrote yesterday of being knocked down by an illness. It has carried over into this day, although with notably less power.

I still am feeling weak and having difficulty concentrating. I am glad to say, however, that the horrendous shivering has departed.

I made my weekly visit to my counselor today and was told I was in heavy ketosis. This, apparently, was decided by the rich color of the urine test strip I produced.

So, I was instructed to add some vegetables to my "normal" meal. I should be happy about that.

It is hard, though. I have no appetite for food right now. So, I am unable to get too excited about that change.

And, I am left to wonder whether my temporary illness has caused the change in calorie-burning speed.

I should be happy about that. It is hard, though.

Day: #*65*   Weight: *179.²*

Food & Water

7:00 a.m.	cappuccino	5:00 p.m.	pill (2nd B-12)
9:00 a.m.	pills (1st B-12)	7:00 p.m.	3rd water done
10:00 a.m.	chocolate bar	7:30 p.m.	ground chicken,
11:45 a.m.	1st water done		broccoli, asparagus,
1:30 p.m.	sloppy joe		spinach, lettuce
3:30 p.m.	2nd water done	8:30 p.m.	cappuccino (decaf)
4:30 p.m.	chocolate bar		

Exercise

None today.

Comments

I awoke today pleased to see my scale reading dip past the 180 mark.

It had been teetering within that whole number for more than a few days.

At my weekly visit to my counselor yesterday, she said my ketosis was "heavy" so an adjustment was necessary.

I was told to add some green vegetables to my main meal. I can say I did that with no objections.

It is nice having that little extra.

I also am quite thrilled to be clear of the illness that struck

...I am functioning like a human again.

me hard yesterday. It has moved elsewhere and I am functioning like a human again.

If good weight equals good health and fewer attacks by such sickness, I am sold. I will continue to work at it just for that alone.

91

Day: #*66*   Weight: *179.*⁴

Food & Water

7:00 a.m.	cappuccino		6:45 p.m.	3rd water done
8:30 a.m.	pills (1st B-12)		7:30 p.m.	salmon, broccoli
10:15 a.m.	1st water done		9:30 p.m.	cappuccino (decaf)
1:15 p.m.	sloppy joe			
2:00 p.m.	2nd water done			
4:15 p.m.	chocolate bar			
4:20 p.m.	pill (2nd B-12)			

Exercise

None today.

Comments

I began this day with little thought to my actual weight. I just got going on my routine. That is good.

Throughout the day, however, I did have at least a couple of occasions when I questioned my stamina for the full tour.

I mean I am getting a bit worn. I have passed the two-month mark and, according to plan, have many more to go.

I really want and need to succeed at this to get my body in shape. But I do need to eat an actual meal again.

There needs to be a new normal, something beyond the packaged meals.

I am nearly halfway home by weight goal but not even a third of the way by expected time in the plan.

So, how will this play out? I will put my head down and press on, but I wonder if I can make it all the way.

There needs to be a new normal...

Day: #*67*   Weight: *178.²*

Food & Water

7:00 a.m.	cappuccino	6:30 p.m.	2nd water done
8:00 a.m.	pills (1st B-12)	7:30 p.m.	ground chicken,
11:00 a.m.	chocolate bar		broccoli, asparagus,
12:00 p.m.	1st water done		spinach, lettuce
1:15 p.m.	chocolate bar	8:00 p.m.	3rd water done
4:15 p.m.	sloppy joe	9:30 p.m.	cappuccino (decaf)
4:50 p.m.	pill (2nd B-12)		

Exercise

None today.

Comments

Weight loss continues, of course.

What made my morning so interesting, however, was what I saw in the shower.

It was clear to me that my legs are visibly thinner. That may sound insignificant. But it took me an extremely long time to recognize they were too hefty.

Seriously, my ankles, calves and thighs are obviously trimmer. They are looking much more normal.

The puffy, inflated look is gone. I am happy about that.

Now, to continue ridding

> *What made my morning interesting, however, is what I saw in the shower.*

my midsection of the extraneous flab... and to build muscle in all the right spots.

I am enthused. Progress—the visible kind—is a great motivator.

Day: **#68**   Weight: **177.⁸**

Food & Water

7:15 a.m.	cappuccino
9:00 a.m.	pills (1st B-12)
10:15 a.m.	chocolate bar
12:00 p.m.	1st water done
1:15 p.m.	chocolate bar
2:30 p.m.	2nd water done
4:15 p.m.	pill (2nd B-12)

4:30 p.m.	sloppy joe
5:30 p.m.	3rd water done
8:00 p.m.	ground chicken, lettuce, spinach, broccoli
10:15 p.m.	cappuccino (decaf)

Exercise

None today.

Comments

My body has made a very visible change and the future will adjust that description to 'radical' change.

It is Saturday, but my dog doesn't understand why that is different from a weekday.

So, she insisted I get up early and set her a plate at the doggy table.

The process got me to the scale for some welcome news, another drop in weight.

I am a few tenths of a pound away from reaching the 30-pound loss mark.

My body has made a very visible change and the future will adjust that description to "radical" change.

So, all is well as I enter another day of my diet program.

94

Day: #*69*   Weight: *177.⁰*

Food & Water

8:30 a.m.	cappuccino
10:15 a.m.	pills (1st B-12)
11:15 a.m.	chocolate bar
12:45 p.m.	1st water done
2:30 p.m.	sloppy joe
2:45 p.m.	2nd water done
5:00 p.m.	chocolate bar
6:30 p.m.	3rd water done
7:45 p.m.	shrimp, scallops, lobster, lettuce, spinach
8:30 p.m.	pill (2nd B-12)
9:00 p.m.	cappuccino (decaf)

Exercise

None today.

Comments

Doing a lot of work around the house today.

I broke up old furniture, loaded it all onto my truck and hauled it to the dump.

It was quite a workout. I am wondering whether I should mark it down as exercise and add some protein to my "normal" meal to compensate.

I have a few hours to go before I sit down to the main meal, so I have some time to decide, or work some more and remove any doubt.

Tonight, for the first time since I began this diet program, I had shellfish as the protein for my "normal" meal.

It was so awesome that I must do it again—maybe many more times!

It was quite a workout. I am wondering whether I should mark it down as exercise...

Day: #*70*   Weight: *177.⁰*

Food & Water

7:00 a.m.	cappuccino		4:20 p.m.	3rd water done
8:00 a.m.	pills (1st B-12)		7:00 p.m.	chicken, broccoli,
11:00 a.m.	chocolate bar			lettuce, spinach
11:30 a.m.	1st water done		7:30 p.m.	pill (2nd B-12)
1:30 p.m.	2nd water done		8:00 p.m.	cappuccino (decaf)
1:45 p.m.	sloppy joe		8:45 p.m.	4th water done
4:15 p.m.	chocolate bar			

Exercise

None today.

Comments

I spent much of my workday preoccupied about the size and fit of my clothes.

I am continuing to shrink and my pants refuse to stay up. That I have my belt latched at the last hole has helped little.

I don't mind buying new britches, but I don't have a lot of time available for such frequent trips to the clothing store.

Also, I am still losing pounds, so, I'll need to get new pants again soon, anyway.

I am not complaining. I am just saying I cannot avoid my mind's focus on the subject.

I am happy with my progress.

I still ain't pretty, but I look way better than I did three months ago.

I am pleased with how I am shaping down.

Don't misunderstand, though. I still ain't pretty, but I look way better than I did three months ago.

96

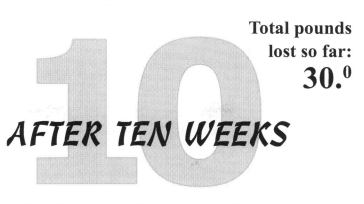

AFTER TEN WEEKS

IMPRESSIONS & PROGRESS

A highlight of this week was my discovery of visible thinness in my body.

I took note of my ankles, calves and thighs being significantly more narrow in their appearance.

I realize that this may seem a small item to others. For me, however, it was a revelation. I had not noticed that they were too bloated before.

Seeing my legs with much more definition and contour had a deep effect on my mental attitude.

The shrinking was a clear sign of success and a reminder that such poor condition can creep up on you without fanfare.

I will be more vigilant in the future by weighing myself every day, even when I am not dieting. Weight must be constantly monitored.

A great benefit of such visible change is how it motivates one to forge ahead happily on the path to good health and fitness.

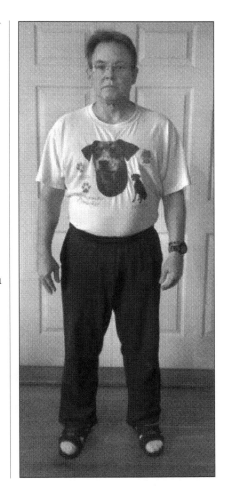

Day: #*71* Weight: *176.⁰*

Food & Water

7:00 a.m.	cappuccino
8:00 a.m.	pills (1st B-12)
10:00 a.m.	chocolate bar
11:00 a.m.	1st water done
12:30 p.m.	sloppy joe
12:45 p.m.	2nd water done
3:30 p.m.	chocolate bar

3:40 p.m.	pill (2nd B-12)
4:30 p.m.	3rd water done
7:30 p.m.	ground chicken, lettuce, spinach, broccoli
8:30 p.m.	cappuccino (decaf)

Exercise

None today.

Comments

Today's weight is precisely 31 pounds below my beginning scale reading.

That is officially my halfway point, I think. In honor of the occasion, I spent a good amount of time daydreaming about reaching my goal weight.

More specifically, I was envisioning how I will look when I have lost the full 62 pounds.

I will not only be much lighter. I will have much greater flexibility and energy. Those improved traits will aid me in my sporting endeavors.

I will not use my new abilities to try to win any competitions. I will just enjoy my outings all the more with a better body.

Ah, yes, almost there. Just have to keep plugging away and enjoying the food.

I will not use my new abilities to try to win any competitions.

98

Day: #*72*   Weight: *175.⁶*

Food & Water

7:00 a.m.	cappuccino
8:30 a.m.	pills (1st B-12)
10:00 a.m.	chocolate bar
10:15 a.m.	1st water done
12:45 p.m.	oatmeal, maple
1:00 p.m.	pill (2nd B-12)
2:00 p.m.	2nd water done
3:30 p.m.	chocolate bar
5:00 p.m.	3rd water done
7:30 p.m.	talapia, broccoli, lettuce
8:00 p.m.	4th water done
9:00 p.m.	chocolate pudding

Exercise

Weights: bench press, 3 sets; military press, 3 sets; curls (bar), 3 sets; curls (dumbs) 3 sets.

Comments

On two separate occasions at work today, people complimented me on how successful I have been on my diet.

All I could say was, "It's pretty easy. All I do is eat the designated food— six times a day— and the weight (fat) goes away."

It was nice to know that people are noticing. I also had a discussion with a friend about the people who are hawking some other diet programs.

In one case, a guy who does advertisements for a national sandwich shop chain lost more than 100 pounds.

Unfortunately, he looks like he still hasn't figured out how to exercise. His look makes me call him "Droopy."

In another case, a singing sensation from the 70s fronts for a national diet program.

She says she lost 50 pounds. I am afraid she has another 20 or 30 to go. She wears black to hide her figure in dim light.

I applaud both of them for dropping significant weight and improving their health.

I plan to surpass their accomplishments, however, and get all the way into great shape.

Day: #*73*   Weight: *175.*⁸

Food & Water

7:00 a.m.	cappuccino
7:45 a.m.	pills (1st B-12)
10:00 a.m.	chocolate bar
10:15 a.m.	1st water done
1:00 p.m.	oatmeal, maple
2:00 p.m.	pill (2nd B-12)
3:45 p.m.	2nd water done

4:00 p.m.	chocolate bar
6:30 p.m.	3rd water done
8:00 p.m.	ground turkey, spinach, broccoli
9:00 p.m.	cappuccino (decaf)

Exercise

None today.

Comments

No weight loss to report today. There was another food incident at work, though.

There was an event yesterday at the office and it was catered by a heavily favored barbeque joint.

I walked into the lounge and a long countertop was invisible under the spread of leftovers.

It was a feast fit for fat folks. I noted that they really could have used help from the old me to make all that chicken and pulled pork vanish quickly.

Now, I said, the best I can do is take some home to the family so it doesn't get wasted.

To throw any of that away would be quite sad... and a shame, since the smell of the sauce was almost enough to make me float off the ground to follow the aroma.

Really, the scent was incredible. It reminded me that one day I will enjoy such food again.

It was a feast fit for fat folks.

Day: #*74*   Weight: *175.⁶*

Food & Water

7:00 a.m.	cappuccino
8:00 a.m.	pills (1st B-12)
10:15 a.m.	chocolate bar
12:45 p.m.	1st water done
1:30 p.m.	sloppy joe
4:20 p.m.	chocolate bar
5:00 p.m.	pill (2nd B-12)
5:05 p.m.	2nd water done
7:30 p.m.	shrimp, lobster, lettuce, spinach, zucchini
8:30 p.m.	cappuccino (decaf)
9:00 p.m.	3rd water done

Exercise

None today.

Comments

I have been having some bothersome back pain today. I have no idea what could be causing it.

I have done nothing physical that would seem to have strained it. So, it makes me wonder whether it is my kidneys acting up.

I have had similar pain during a previous diet when my carbohydrate intake was reduced to nearly none.

Since I eat a suitable amount of carbohydrates on this program, I am ruling out that cause.

That leaves me with no answer and no suspicions. I am at a loss.

That leaves me with no answers and no suspicions.

I can confirm the pain is real, however. I can only hope at this point that a good night's sleep will send the pain packing.

I will know more in the morning.

Day: #*75*   Weight: *175.⁰*

Food & Water

7:45 a.m.	cappuccino		6:00 p.m.	3rd water done
8:30 a.m.	pills (1st B-12)		8:30 p.m.	ground chicken, lettuce, spinach, broccoli
11:00 a.m.	chocolate bar			
11:30 a.m.	1st water done			
2:00 p.m.	macaroni & cheese		9:30 p.m.	chocolate pudding
2:00 p.m.	pill (2nd B-12)		11:00 p.m.	cappuccino (decaf)
3:15 p.m.	2nd water done			

Exercise

Run: 15 minutes (w/dog).

Comments

Ah, relief. I woke up and my back pain was gone. I still am unable to pinpoint the cause, but I will settle for not feeling that discomfort.

I also have been having on-and-off trouble with an ankle. It became "pain on" during my run today.

The thing has swelled a bit and is making it difficult for me to walk normally.

I must limp to keep from putting too much weight on that side.

I don't know what is causing the trouble. But I think the longer I am kind to it the less likely it will flare up and the greater the chance it will heal and stop being an issue.

So, I suppose I will be swimming more and pounding the pavement less.

I must limp to keep from putting too much weight on that side.

Day: #*76*   Weight: *174.*²

Food & Water

8:45 a.m.	cappuccino
9:45 a.m.	pills (1st B-12)
11:30 a.m.	1st water done
11:45 a.m.	chocolate bar
3:15 p.m.	2nd water done
3:30 p.m.	beef/veggie soup
5:15 p.m.	3rd water done

7:30 p.m.	beef, broccoli, lettuce, spinach, mashed potatoes
7:45 p.m.	pill (2nd B-12)
8:00 p.m.	4th water done
8:30 p.m.	cappuccino (decaf)

Exercise

None today.

Comments

My ankle is feeling a lot better today, although I will refrain from running on it for a while.

My wife and I have been discussing whether the difficulty could be associated with a circulation issue.

I believe that is not the case. I am unable to rule anything out, but the ankle pain is not a muscle problem. It seems to be a joint-tendon matter.

When I had muscle cramps, they were attributed to a need for more water and dark green leafy vegetables to aid blood flow.

I took those corrective actions and seem to have fixed

I believe that is not the case. I am unable to rule anything out, but...

that problem. I believe if I avoid running on my ankle for a while, it will have time to recover and I will be fine.

We shall see.

Day: #77   Weight: *174.*⁴

Food & Water

7:45 a.m.   cappuccino
8:10 a.m.   pills (1st B-12)
10:45 a.m. chocolate bar
11:30 a.m. 1st water done
1:45 p.m.   oatmeal, maple
4:45 p.m.   chocolate bar
5:00 p.m.   2nd water done

7:30 p.m.   chicken, lettuce,
            broccoli
8:00 p.m.   cappuccino (decaf)
8:45 p.m.   pill (2nd B-12)
9:00 p.m.   3rd water done

Exercise

None today.

Comments

I did plenty of walking today. We were shopping, a trip that took us to several stores.

By the end, my ankle was quite sore. It is clear I will be unable to run for some time.

I got some relief from an elastic brace we bought that stretches over the foot and up the leg a bit.

Still, I must pamper it until it heals.

The notable event of the day was when, in a discussion with the wife, I read a laundry list of my favorite restaurants and my special dish at each and how I would enjoy them all again one day after

I have completed this program.

Well, I had to back pedal a bit. I don't mean I will return to my old, horrible ways of eating.

I will partake in the favorite delights only occasionally. And I will limit the amount of food at each setting, too.

It also should be mentioned that my reminiscing should not be confused with unwanted "cravings."

It was just a normal stroll down memory lane.

11

**Total pounds
lost so far:
32.⁶**

AFTER ELEVEN WEEKS

IMPRESSIONS & PROGRESS

The positive aspects of this past week include several instances when I visualized my new appearance, the look I will have when I reach my goal weight.

I suppose this mental activity also can accomplish many benefits outside of the diet program in which I am participating. It seems to be particularly useful in this scenario, however.

When you combine it with the success I have achieved so far, it serves as an assistant catalyst. It is the basis of a renewed enthusiasm on my part.

It helps me to forge ahead and jump into exercise with vigor. It also allowed me to power through a few office parties without reaching for calorie-laden junk food spread out for the taking.

Never again will I underestimate the value of visualization.

I just need to remember to call on this approach more often.

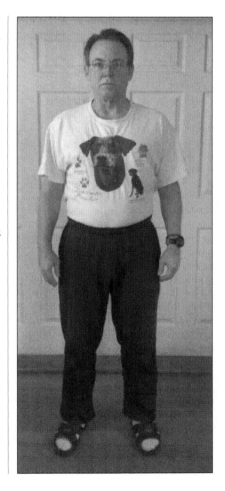

Day: #*78*   Weight: *173.*^8

Food & Water

7:15 a.m.	cappuccino
9:00 a.m.	pills (1st B-12)
10:15 a.m.	chocolate bar
11:00 a.m.	1st water done
1:15 p.m.	oatmeal, maple
2:45 p.m.	pill (2nd B-12)
3:30 p.m.	2nd water done

4:05 p.m.	chocolate bar
7:30 p.m.	ground chicken, lettuce, broccoli
8:30 p.m.	cappuccino (decaf)
9:00 p.m.	3rd water done

Exercise

None today.

Comments

Today was my weekly visit with my counselor. There is nothing special to report.

Wait. I lost 3½ pounds this past week. That is above the average and I am thrilled.

Other than that, everything was just normal, my blood pressure, included.

I stayed busy enough at work that I didn't have time to think about my diet. I had to force myself to remember to eat, drink and take pills at the right times.

When work was through, I did fall back to the thought pattern that swirls around the length of the program.

If I project a two-pounds-per-week average loss, that leaves me with about 15 more weeks to go.

That accounts for no lengthy plateaus or other delays, and still, that is almost four months.

It only has been a little more than two so far and I am ready to be done.

I am not suffering. I just want to get to my goal pretty soon.

Day: #*79*   Weight: *174.*²

Food & Water

7:30 a.m.	cappuccino	5:30 p.m.	2nd water done
8:15 a.m.	pills (1st B-12)	7:00 p.m.	beef, broccoli,
10:15 a.m.	1st water done		lettuce,
10:30 a.m.	chocolate bar	7:45 p.m.	cappuccino (decaf)
1:00 p.m.	oatmeal, maple	10:30 p.m.	3rd water done
1:15 p.m.	pill (2nd B-12)		
4:30 p.m.	chocolate bar		

Exercise

None today.

Comments

Today held no major excitements, no heavy pains, no notable achievements.

The only thing to mention was an extended period of time between meals.

I was stuck in a drawn-out meeting that kept me from my chocolate bar.

I normally spread my meals out to avoid gaps because my day is fairly long.

I am up at 6 a.m. and off to work. I am usually home at 5 p.m. or so, but I have duties involving six-year-old twins.

There are baths, dinner and homework. So, my last consumption comes around 10 p.m., if I wait.

The meeting kept me more than an hour-and-a-half beyond my scheduled snack time.

I was understandably a bit hungry by the time my teeth found their way into that tasty morsel.

Day: #*80*   Weight: *173.⁶*

Food & Water

7:00 a.m.	cappuccino		4:15 p.m.	chocolate bar
8:15 a.m.	pills (1st B-12)		7:30 p.m.	talapia, spinach, lettuce, broccoli
10:00 a.m.	chocolate bar			
10:30 a.m.	1st water done		8:30 p.m.	cappuccino (decaf)
1:15 p.m.	soup, chicken/rice		9:00 p.m.	3rd water done
1:30 p.m.	pill (2nd B-12)			
3:30 p.m.	2nd water done			

Exercise

None today.

Comments

My thoughts today center around my weight. That can be no surprise. But I could have said, "centered around my waist."

That is because I have achieved a weight that seems very normal. I mean that I believe many, if not most, people would consider my current body situation a success.

I have lost more than 30 pounds and my shape has improved drastically.

I can move among the crowds and fit in well. I mean "blend" in well.

I do not appear to be heavy while I am mingling with the public. I do want to take this program to its proposed end, however.

I don't want to stop at "average." I want to arrive at "ideal" weight for my gender and height.

I can do it. I just need to remain patient and press onward.

I am still losing pounds. No need to think of quitting yet.

Charge!

Day: #*81*   Weight: *173.*⁶

Food & Water

8:00 a.m.	cappuccino
9:00 a.m.	pills (1st B-12)
11:00 a.m.	chocolate bar
11:15 a.m.	1st water done
2:00 p.m.	oatmeal, maple
2:15 p.m.	pill (2nd B-12)
3:00 p.m.	2nd water done

4:30 p.m.	3rd water done
4:45 p.m.	chocolate bar
8:00 p.m.	lobster, scallops, broccoli, lettuce, spinach
9:00 p.m.	cappuccino (decaf)

Exercise

None today.

Comments

The instructions were pretty clear. I confirmed this by glancing at them after the disaster.

The package had the necessary info on the back. It said, "4 to 6 ounces of water."

Nothing in those numbers and words should make a person see or think of "eight."

But, I poured that excessive amount into my bowl of oatmeal.

Of course, it was just enough liquid to ensure that the concoction never would resemble its intended form.

Even boiling it down was unable to transform it beyond soup.

It also could be described as a maple and brown sugar puddle. So, what to do?

I could scrap it, eat a chocolate bar for this meal and get a replacement later at home.

Or, I could toughen up, grab a soup spoon and make it disappear, checking off that meal without wasting the cost of that purchase.

I don't want to brag, but...

Day: #*82*   Weight: *172.*⁶

Food & Water

8:15 a.m.   cappuccino
9:00 a.m.   pills (1st B-12)
10:45 a.m. 1st water done
11:00 a.m. chocolate bar
12:15 p.m. 2nd water done
3:00 p.m.   3rd water done
3:15 p.m.   soup, chicken/rice

5:30 p.m.   chocolate bar
9:30 p.m.   pork, spinach,
            lettuce, broccoli
9:45 p.m.   pill (2nd B-12)
10:00 p.m. cappuccino (decaf)

Exercise

None today.

Comments

I discovered a couple of things. I forgot to bring my big blue bottle to work with me, so I had to drink store-bought bottled water that I had stashed near my desk.

I realized that drinking water at room temperature made it go down much faster.

Also, not having it iced kept me from feeling cold all day. That was a big improvement.

The other thing worth noting was my experience with tea.

Now, I am sure everyone who is a fan of tea is waiting to hear what odd thing occurred.

Well, nothing strange took place. I just realized that I like it a lot and can drink plenty of it on this diet program because it has a negligible amount of calories.

After soaking the tea bag in a cup of steaming hot water, I add an artificial sweetener to enhance the flavor.

That is another way to warm my innards (now that I have less insulating fat on my outer shell) and it makes me happy.

Day: #*83*   Weight: *171.*⁸

Day: #*83*   Weight: $171.^{8}$

Food & Water

9:15 a.m.	cappuccino	7:30 p.m.	chicken, lettuce
10:00 a.m.	pills (1st B-12)	9:30 p.m.	4th water done
11:45 a.m.	1st water done	10:00 p.m.	chocolate pudding
12:15 p.m.	soup, chicken/rice	10:15 p.m.	pill (2nd B-12)
12:30 p.m.	2nd water done	10:30 p.m.	cappuccino (decaf)
3:30 p.m.	chocolate bar		
3:45 p.m.	3rd water done		

Exercise

Weights: bench press, 3 sets; military press, 3 sets; curls (bar), 3 sets; curls (dumbs), 3 sets; squats, 3 sets.

Comments

I made another discovery today. I slung my weight belt around my waist, threaded the end through the buckle, wrenched it snug and found that I had shrunk a full two notches.

Yes, that is two sizes. I don't know how I missed the one in between.

I haven't been away from lifting all that long. I would not have been shocked to learn of a single-notch move. A double jump, however, caught me by surprise.

This diet program keeps offering up these tidbits of evidence of success. There is a steady stream of things that put a smile on my face.

I would not have been shocked to learn of a single-notch move.
A double jump, however...

Day: #*84*   Weight: *171.⁸*

Food & Water

8:15 a.m.	cappuccino
8:45 a.m.	pills (1st B-12)
10:00 a.m.	1st water done
11:15 a.m.	chocolate bar
1:45 p.m.	2nd water done
2:15 p.m.	chocolate bar
7:15 p.m.	3rd water done

7:30 p.m.	ground chicken, lettuce, broccoli, spinach
8:00 p.m.	cappuccino (decaf)
8:15 p.m.	pill (2nd B-12)
9:00 p.m.	chocolate shake

Exercise

None today.

Comments

I don't know what the rest of the day might bring. This morning, however, I am impressed enough with my current status to begin writing.

At this moment, I am feeling quite happy. The kids are at home because of a school break. I can hear them playing in the next room.

I have a warm feeling inside. Some of it is attributable to my happy kids. The rest is caused by a couple of cups of hot tea.

I am sure all of this is directly connected to my diet program because I have lost so much unwanted fat so far.

Back when I was obese, I was so easily irritated.

Nowadays, I am calm enough to thoroughly enjoy the simpler things in life. And I think I will pack up the family and go to a local park to get some sunshine and let the kids run and play.

The latter activity is seeming like a necessity now.

The kids have turned on each other. The vicious verbal barbs require a suitable intervention.

Off we go.

12

AFTER TWELVE WEEKS

IMPRESSIONS & PROGRESS

Another successful week goes into the record book.

I weighed in at three-and-a-half pounds less than the week before at my regularly scheduled appointment.

That may be my largest drop since the initial dip of the first two weeks. I would like to continue this pace. It would help me finish a bit earlier than planned.

Having dropped 35 pounds, I now am an "average" weight. This seems to be where lots of people stop. I am determined to get to ideal weight, however.

I made a couple of discoveries in the past week. One, I can drink more water faster if I take it at room temperature. Two, hot tea is calorie-free flavored water that warms me inside and helps me get through the day.

My lower weight has aided my mental attitude, too. I am much calmer in all aspects of life. And that is a great reward in itself.

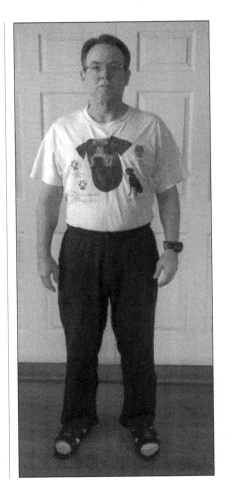

5

Thankful for less fat and a lot more

*W*ow! The period just completed included the biggest, most celebrated meal of the year: Thanksgiving. I am pleased to inform that I breezed through it without a struggle.

While I have spent a life enjoying the turkey, stuffing, mashed potatoes and pumpkin pie like the rest of the country, my desire to stay on track with my diet ruled the day.

I must confess that all the eating was not missed. The important aspects of the holiday remained and were enjoyed.

I spent the day in the company of family. We even sat down to a traditional dinner together. They had all the "fixings" and I ate my "normal" meal.

I had ground chicken and proper vegetables. My food tasted excellent and was quite sufficient in bulk, since I set my mind right from the beginning.

I prepared by focusing on my spouse and children and telling myself the food of the day was irrelevant.

I suppose that is a lesson by which to live. Food should be a thing we consume to sustain life.

The flavors and thrill of devouring them should not be a driving force in our existence.

That lifestyle ensures that we will be overweight constantly. When meals are merely maintenance, we easily can control our weight and have a positive effect on our health.

The period also was significant because I saw a noticeable change to my body's shape and the size of its parts.

Of course, if you never have experienced such a thing yet, you would think it is no big deal.

I must point out, however, that the brain has the ability to mask reality. That is why I never really understood how far into obesity I had stumbled.

When I gazed into a mirror, I saw only an average-weight person staring back at me. It seemed to be mental and visual rationalization.

So, if I was unable to see how bad my body had gotten, it should be no surprise that it took drastic size reduction for the alteration to become visible in the eyes that send images to a protective brain.

I believe I can see more clearly now. I also am vowing to be very critical when I examine my weight and body condition in the future.

I will trust the scale and tape measure to tell the true tale of my situation. The mirror will be held in contempt and used only as a necessary evil in the search for lengthy whiskers or unwanted sun-scorched blemishes that suggest further inspection by a professional is needed.

Thus, the visual discovery

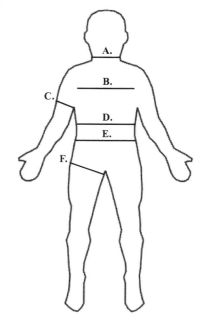

A. Neck: 15.^{5}

B. Chest: 42.^{5}

C. Biceps: 13

D. Waist (navel): 37.^{5}

E. High Hip (belt line): 36.^{5}

F. Thighs: 22.^{5}

G. Weight: 171.^{8}

turned out to be an extremely valuable lesson to remember long after my diet is done.

Another pleasant result of dieting realized during this past period was a psychological calm that was difficult, if not impossible, to obtain previously.

Without conscious effort, I remained relaxed in situations that once had made me severely grumpy.

It was my wife who first noticed this change. She was pleased to welcome my new attitude.

I am unable to explain it, since I really had no knowledge of my fat-induced irritability.

Even as a distant observer, however, I can say that a sense of calm at all times is a most welcome characteristic.

It will pay great dividends to anyone who has mastered the art of controlling one's mind and actions.

I will conclude this section with another discovery that was far less significant than the others I have noted. It is, nonetheless, worth mentioning.

The program's requirement to drink at least 60 ounces of water each day made me a little anxious.

I am not much of a plain water drinker. Diet cola was my beverage of habit. So, I decided that water would be fine, if I smothered it in ice.

It worked. I enjoyed it much more than expected. One day, however, ice was unobtainable. I had to drink the liquid at room temperature. Well, it actually was a blessing. The ice-free water went down faster and more smoothly.

It caused no shock to the throat. So, that is how I continue to consume the necessary quantities.

This method is not unenjoyable and it is a much more efficient way to arrive at the appropriate level of hydration.

All I can say is, "Try it!"

Day: #*85*   Weight: *171.*⁶

Food & Water

8:30 a.m.	cappuccino
9:00 a.m.	pills (1st B-12)
11:15 a.m.	chocolate bar
11:30 a.m.	1st water done
2:15 p.m.	soup, chicken/rice
2:30 p.m.	2nd water done
5:15 p.m.	chocolate bar

8:00 p.m.	ground chicken, lettuce, broccoli, spinach
8:30 p.m.	cappuccino (decaf)
9:40 p.m.	3rd water done

Exercise

None today.

Comments

Today I nearly forgot I was on a diet. Not that I was eating badly. I am way too dedicated for that.

I mean that I am on vacation from work and I was very casual in my activities. I mostly stayed at the house... I watched an old favorite movie. I went out to run an errand and had my appointment with my diet counselor.

As I reach the advanced stages of my program, there is very little to be achieved in our meetings.

I hop onto the scale, of course. She records the number. She takes my blood pressure and asks if I have any questions.

That is about it on days when the analyzer has no part of my visit.

I am not complaining about the brevity of our sessions. I am pointing out that we are on "cruise control."

Everything is progressing according to plan. And seeing a knowledgeable nutritionist is an extremely valuable part of the program.

That expertise is a main reason I chose this program over the many others that are available.

I like being monitored and held accountable.

Day: #*86*   Weight: *172.⁰*

Food & Water

9:00 a.m.	cappuccino
10:00 a.m.	pills (1st B-12)
12:05 p.m.	chocolate bar
12:10 p.m.	1st water done
3:30 p.m.	soup, chicken/rice
6:15 p.m.	2nd water done
6:20 p.m.	pill (2nd B-12)

7:30 p.m.	steak, lettuce, broccoli, spinach
7:45 p.m.	3rd water done
8:15 p.m.	cappuccino (decaf)
8:30 p.m.	chocolate bar

Exercise

None today.

Comments

I had planned for a pretty lazy day. The only stressful interruption would be a nice lap-swimming session at a nearby community pool.

I packed up the kids and sent them off to the park with their friends and an adult chaperone.

I drove at a leisurely pace for the two miles or so to arrive at my destination.

I found the parking lot nearly empty. Hmm, I thought. I am either going to have the pool to myself... or the place is closed today.

I put the buggy in gear and thought about other ways to properly exert myself. I came up with nothing.

Before I could remember I wanted to watch a movie, the kids burst through the door and chattered at eardrum-piercing sound levels.

So, my highlight of the day was a bowl of chicken and rice soup (with spice added) courtesy of my diet plan.

This selection is one of the most filling items on the shelf and one of my favorites. It requires the addition of at least salt and pepper, however; otherwise, it is far too bland.

Day: #*87*   Weight: *171.²*

Food & Water

8:15 a.m.	cappuccino		broccoli, spinach
9:00 a.m.	pills (1st B-12)	7:00 p.m.	cappuccino (decaf)
11:30 a.m.	chocolate bar	7:15 p.m.	pill (2nd B-12)
1:45 p.m.	1st water done	9:30 p.m.	oatmeal, maple
3:00 p.m.	soup, chicken/rice	10:00 p.m.	3rd water done
5:00 p.m.	2nd water done		
6:30 p.m.	turkey, lettuce,		

Exercise

None today.

Comments

Today is Christmas. In the preceding days, I was asked several times whether I would have difficulty at the holiday meal. Even my diet counselor seemed concerned.

I waived it all off. I have been rock solid from the beginning. I have not swayed from my designated path by even one bite of forbidden food.

I know the fastest route to my goal will result from strict adherence to the plan, So, it was a bit surprising when I found myself looking over the long table of foods, a variety that was most inviting.

I had no urge to jump in and gobble enormous quantities. No, I just felt a bit deprived because I couldn't even have a taste of the delicious foods everyone at the table was raving about.

Oh, well, I survived. When I arrive at thin and healthy, I will know such refrain was well worth the trouble.

Oh, well, I survived.

120

Day: #*88*   Weight: *171.⁴*

Food & Water

8:45 a.m.	cappuccino
9:30 a.m.	pills (1st B-12)
11:30 a.m.	chocolate bar
1:30 p.m.	1st water done
2:30 p.m.	chocolate bar
3:00 p.m.	2nd water done
7:45 p.m.	ground chicken,

broccoli, lettuce, spinach

8:15 p.m.	cappuccino (decaf)
8:30 p.m.	pill (2nd B-12)
8:45 p.m.	3rd water done
9:30 p.m.	soup, chicken/rice

Exercise

None today.

Comments

My weight was up two-tenths of a pound at this morning's scale mounting.

I know that is no big amount. It comes, however, after a couple or three days of flatlining—no drop. So, I am wondering if I should begin to get concerned.

I don't want to have come all this way only to stall out as I near the finish line.

I want nothing to interfere with my success. I want nary a single day's delay.

I am not being greedy. This program is a change in lifestyle that seems simple—and it is—in the short term. But for a long

I want nary a single day's delay.

haul, several months, it does become a job with an end goal.

I am hoping previous plateaus and their remedies (outcomes) will repeat this time. If so, I should see a significant drop tomorrow.

Best of luck to me!

Day: #*89*   Weight: *171.*⁴

Day: #*89*   Weight: *171.*⁴

Food & Water

8:30 a.m.	cappuccino		5:30 p.m.	chocolate bar
8:45 a.m.	pills (1st B-12)		8:30 p.m.	ground chicken,
11:10 a.m.	1st water done			broccoli, lettuce,
11:30 a.m.	chocolate bar			spinach
2:30 p.m.	soup, chicken/rice		9:00 p.m.	cappuccino (decaf)
3:00 p.m.	2nd water done		10:00 p.m.	3rd water done
3:15 p.m.	pill (2nd B-12)			

Exercise

None today.

Comments

I am stuck. Today's weight is the same as yesterday. This makes about four days without a drop.

My only hope is that a jaw-dropping reduction is imminent. That would wash away the bad feeling I have from this poor trend.

I will get no hopes up.

I gave no thought to my weight the rest of the day. I did lots of things with the kids. That was much more productive than worrying about my next scale reading.

I am going to bed, however, and, contrary to my own advice, I have big hopes for a vast improvement by morning. We

That was much more productive than worrying about my next scale reading.

shall see.

Maybe a good dream about being very fit and thin will give a boost to my chances.

Day: #*90*   Weight: *171.⁰*

Food & Water

8:00 a.m.	cappuccino
9:00 a.m.	pills (1st B-12)
10:30 a.m.	1st water done
11:15 a.m.	oatmeal, maple
2:30 p.m.	soup, chicken/rice
3:00 p.m.	2nd water done
3:05 p.m.	pill (2nd B-12)

5:45 p.m.	chocolate bar
7:00 p.m.	3rd water done
7:30 p.m.	ground chicken, lettuce, broccoli, zucchini
8:00 p.m.	chocolate pudding
9:00 p.m.	4th water done

Exercise

Weights: bench press, 3 sets; military press, 3 sets; curls (bar), 3 sets.

Comments

So, there is still time for the scale to respond appropriately before then.

Well, I had no drastic drop in weight this morning. So, as I glance back at my records, I see it has taken about seven days to crush just one pound of fat into oblivion.

That is not an acceptable pace. I don't know what is causing the slow going. My appointment with my counselor is two days away.

So, there is still time for the scale to respond appropriately before then.

If not, or even if so, it will be an opportunity to compare our records, since we are not exactly aligned.

123

Day: #*91*   Weight: *170.*⁸

Food & Water

8:30 a.m.	cappuccino
9:30 a.m.	pills (1st B-12)
11:45 a.m.	soup, chicken/rice
12:10 p.m.	1st water done
1:15 p.m.	2nd water done
2:30 p.m.	chocolate bar
2:45 p.m.	3rd water done

6:00 p.m.	chocolate bar
7:30 p.m.	steak, lettuce, broccoli
8:00 p.m.	pill (2nd B-12)
8:15 p.m.	cappuccino (decaf)
9:30 p.m.	4th water done

Exercise

None today.

Comments

I just felt like I wanted a bite of pumpkin pie, a shrimp taco, a nice pasta.

While we were out and about, I had several separate thoughts of meals at a variety of restaurants. I also had thoughts of other foods while shopping in the grocery store.

I have no explanation. I was not feeling overly hungry at the time. I just felt like I wanted a bite of pumpkin pie, a shrimp taco, a nice pasta.

But I am back at home and about five minutes from my diet's packaged meal.

I still have little hunger and those bad foods have vanished from my mind. So, I guess I have returned to normal. Good thing!

AFTER THIRTEEN WEEKS

IMPRESSIONS & PROGRESS

This was a one-pound week. How tragic! I am supposed to "keep a stiff lip" and ignore that dismal result, but I am truly bothered by it.

Of course, a significant drop tomorrow morning would erase the mental punishment I have withstood while watching the snail-like pace of the week.

I did have an experience from which I can take a good lesson. I was out shopping and began imagining the restaurant-made and home-cooked meals I have been forsaking for the last few months.

I was not overly hungry at the time. When I got home, however, the thoughts departed without a trace. I ate my packaged meal as scheduled and realized that wandering the aisles of the grocery store probably was the spark that ignited those faint desires.

The environment probably was completely to blame. Exiting it seemed to be the cure.

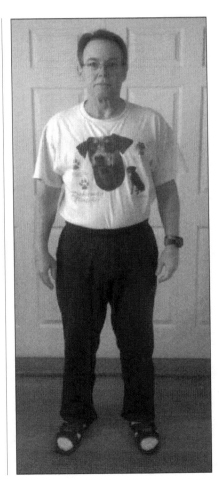

Day: #*92*   Weight: *170.*⁸

Food & Water

8:00 a.m.	cappuccino		6:30 p.m.	soup, chickern/rice
8:30 a.m.	pills (1st B-12)		7:00 p.m.	3rd water done
11:30 a.m.	salmon, broccoli, lettuce		7:30 p.m.	peanut butter soft serve
12:30 p.m.	1st water done		8:15 p.m.	cappuccino (decaf)
3:30 p.m.	chocolate bar			
6:10 p.m.	2nd water done			

Exercise

None today.

Comments

Well, I was not saved by the scale this morning.

There was no significant, last-minute drop in my weight. Thus, it actually was a one-pound week. My visit to meet my diet counselor confirmed this.

There was a twist, however. Proving again why a counselor is so valuable, mine examined my body analysis, created by the computerized scale, and showed me a different perspective.

While it is true the scale only displayed a pound dip below last week's number, that is only part of the story.

I also have been adding muscle, which will burn calories faster. And my measurements also show that I am losing inches in the right places.

Lastly, since I have lost 36 pounds so far, my body is adjusting and will get back on track very soon.

And a slightly slower pace is acceptable.

Because I have heard this all before, I could say, "Yeah, I know that." But it is great to be reminded at precisely the right moment by one of the program's greatest assets.

Day: #*93*   Weight: *169.*^{2}

Food & Water

8:30 a.m.	cappuccino
8:45 a.m.	pills (1st B-12)
11:30 a.m.	oatmeal, maple
12:15 p.m.	1st water done
2:30 p.m.	soup, chicken/rice
3:15 p.m.	2nd water done
5:45 p.m.	chocolate bar

7:30 p.m.	ground chicken, lettuce, broccoli, spinach
8:00 p.m.	cappuccino (decaf)
9:00 p.m.	pill (2nd B-12)

Exercise

Run: 15 minutes w/dog.
Weights: bench press, 3 sets; military press, 3 sets; curls (bar), 3 sets; squats, 3 sets.

Comments

Alas! The game rages on. After a week of the scale getting the better of me, it has collapsed.

Well, it stumbled, at least, by a pound and a half. That was the significant drop I have been awaiting.

I am unable to rest easy, however. More flat spots will come. I must ask myself: why am I no more able to handle them now than when I began this program?

I have weathered at least a few already and felt I had learned the lesson.

Apparently, school is still in session.

Of course, I could avoid this psychological battle by weighing myself but once each week.

I would not see the jagged daily results and, surely, the weekly observation always would show a drop, even if only a slight one.

I justify my daily, curiosity by analogizing it to the numerous other small steps I must take daily—record my meals, pills, exercise, thoughts.

Why should I jettison just one? I think, in the end, I enjoy the jousting with my scale, mostly because I continue to win!

Day: #*94*   Weight: *169.*⁶

Food & Water

8:15 a.m.	cappuccino
8:45 a.m.	pills (1st B-12)
11:00 a.m.	1st water done
11:15 a.m.	soup, chicken/rice
12:00 p.m.	2nd water done
2:00 p.m.	chocolate bar
5:00 p.m.	chocolate bar

7:30 p.m.	ground chicken, broccoli, spinach
8:05 p.m.	3rd water done
9:45 p.m.	pill (2nd B-12)
10:00 p.m.	cappuccino (decaf)

Exercise

None today.

Comments

My weight bounced up a little bit this morning. But, that has little significance.

I am still happy about the pleasant and meaningful drop I experienced yesterday.

The rest of this day was uneventful, as far as the diet is concerned.

I stayed active. We took the kids and our youngest and largest dog to the beach.

We followed that with a trip to the park. The kids rode their bikes, training wheels and all, around a lengthy concrete loop.

These activities are relevant because they consume time and keep me far from the house. As such, I was able to eat on time only because I easily carried my chocolate bars with me.

That is a welcomed convenience.

While I might have preferred a bowl of oatmeal or soup, I had no way to mix and cook those options while I was out and about.

I enjoyed the bars and accomplished the scheduled meals without fanfare.

Day: #95   Weight: *168.*⁶

Food & Water

9:00 a.m.	cappuccino
9:30 a.m.	pills (1st B-12)
12:15 p.m.	oatmeal, maple
1:00 p.m.	1st water done
3:15 p.m.	soup, chicken/rice
3:45 p.m.	2nd water done
6:30 p.m.	pill (2nd B-12)

7:15 p.m.	steak, lettuce, broccoli, zucchini, spinach
7:45 p.m.	3rd water done
8:30 p.m.	soup, chicken/rice
9:30 p.m.	cappuccino (decaf)

Exercise

None today.

Comments

No major events took place today.

My back pain keeps flashing onto me, though, and I have been feeling cold most of the day.

A steady flow of hot tea has been unable to warm me.

It is a type of cold that is deep inside of me, too far from, and unaffected by, a thick coat or heavy sweater.

I will try to remember to ask my counselor about this constant chill.

Maybe it is unrelated to this diet. Maybe my back pain also has nothing to to do with this fat-reduction program. That would be hard to believe, however.

A major loss of weight and significant change of diet almost certainly is connected to the maladies I am experiencing.

It seems especially likely they are all related to each other, since I have no other symptoms that would tell me I am just getting sick.

So, the search for answers continues.

Day: #*96* Weight: *168.*⁴

Weight: $168.^4$

Food & Water

9:00 a.m.	cappuccino		5:30 p.m.	oatmeal, maple
9:30 a.m.	pills (1st B-12)		8:30 p.m.	ground chicken, broccoli, lettuce
9:45 a.m.	1st water done			
12:05 p.m.	soup, chicken/rice		9:15 p.m.	pill (2nd B-12)
12:30 p.m.	2nd water done		9:30 p.m.	4th water done
2:45 p.m.	chocolate bar		10:00 p.m.	cappuccino (decaf)
3:00 p.m.	3rd water done			

Exercise

None today.

Comments

I learned an extremely valuable lesson today.

When I first awoke this morning, I jumped onto the scale as my routine dictates. I was annoyed to see my weight was up two-tenths of a pound from yesterday.

I went back to bed. About 15 minutes later, I got up and headed to the shower.

Out of curiosity, I stepped aboard the scale. The reading was down four-tenths from the number found just minutes earlier.

There were no other variables. Only a little time had passed. I know that scale readings will alter throughout the day, but this episode revealed severe variation only minutes apart.

It helps me understand the true insignificance of a precise scale reading at a particular moment in time.

It reiterates the need to take a poor reading with a "grain of salt," as they say.

It is vital to focus on the bigger picture, the overall trend, or the general area of weight.

130

Day: #*97*   Weight: *169.⁰*

Food & Water

8:45 a.m.	cappuccino
10:00 a.m.	pills (1st B-12)
11:55 a.m.	soup, chicken/rice
12:30 p.m.	1st water done
1:30 p.m.	2nd water done
3:30 p.m.	oatmeal, maple
6:15 p.m.	chocolate bar

7:30 p.m.	shrimp, lettuce, broccoli,
8:00 p.m.	cappuccino (decaf)
8:05 p.m.	pill (2nd B-12)
8:30 p.m.	3rd water done

Exercise

Run: 15 minutes w/dog. Weights: bench press, 3 sets; military press, 3 sets; curls (bar), 3 sets; curls (dumbs), 3 sets; crunches, 25.

Comments

I was on fire for exercise today. My ankle was feeling better. So, I began with a run.

Shortly thereafter, I hit the weights. It felt pretty good. I also added crunches for the first time.

I figured it was time to start tightening my stomach muscles because they will be more visible soon.

The last poundage I need to lose seems concentrated around my belly. The result of crunches also will aid my posture.

Interestingly, later while out shopping, I ran into a married couple I had not seen in a few months.

They complimented me on my new look and inquired about the program. I showered them with info and the wife asked how much exercise was required.

I noted that it is minimal in the beginning, but everyone should develop the habit.

I got the impression they won't be making a call to the program office anytime soon, regardless of how much I stressed the success was nearly effortless.

131

Day: #*98*   Weight: *169.*⁶

Food & Water

7:00 a.m.	cappuccino	5:00 p.m.	2nd water done
8:30 a.m.	pills (1st B-12)	7:30 p.m.	talapia, lettuce,
10:15 a.m.	oatmeal, maple		broccoli
11:00 a.m.	1st water done	8:00 p.m.	3rd water done
1:15 p.m.	chocolate bar	8:15 p.m.	cappuccino (decaf)
4:30 p.m.	pill (2nd B-12)		
4:45 p.m.	soup, chicken/rice		

Exercise

None today.

Comments

My weight was on a slight upswing this morning. It had little effect on my thought processes.

I guess I am used to it. I say that now. But, if it continues to climb, I probably will get riled.

I had some thoughts about self esteem today. I was remembering how I felt when I was large.

I never thought of myself as hideous. I probably should have. Maybe I was in denial.

I do remember having a discussion with a friend about being unable to see the extent of my obesity when I looked into the mirror.

He said, "I think we see what we want to see." I believe he was right.

I remember avoiding allowing photos to be taken of me. Those things always exposed my horrible condition.

I am feeling good about my progress now and I plan to take regular and frequent pictures of my body so I can continue to monitor my status.

It is the only way, since I am unwilling to trust the reflective glass in the bathroom.

14

AFTER FOURTEEN WEEKS

IMPRESSIONS & PROGRESS

I found great frustration this week. I spent many days with the same scale reading. I still am unaccustomed to the flat spots, even thought I know I should ignore them.

My program counselor came to the rescue. She reminded me that just because the scale seems motionless, it may not tell the whole story.

The body can and does continue to burn fat while building muscle. They can offset each other and make a dieter believe no progress is being made, based on the stillness of the scale number.

That was good news to me and it gave me a good feeling. It was a great help to have my mind put back at ease. More than the physical challenges, the mental ping-pong that occurs during a diet program can be the downfall of the weight-loss enthusiast.

Thus, it is imperative to keep the brain happy. Otherwise, disaster and failure can arrive.

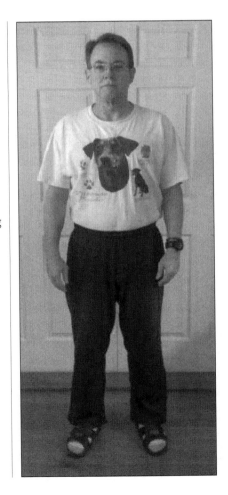

Day: #*99*   Weight: *168.*[8]

Food & Water

7:00 a.m.	cappuccino	4:15 p.m.	chocolate bar
7:30 a.m.	pills (1st B-12)	7:30 p.m.	ground chicken,
10:15 a.m.	oatmeal, maple		lettuce, zucchini
11:00 a.m.	1st water done	8:00 p.m.	cappuccino (decaf)
1:00 p.m.	pill (2nd B-12)	8:30 p.m.	3rd water done
1:15 p.m.	sloppy joe		
3:00 p.m.	2nd water done		

Exercise

None today.

Comments

I had my weekly checkup today at the program office. Surprisingly, despite my observations, I apparently lost almost three pounds this week.

That doesn't mean my readings are wrong. It reflects that our "weeks" are misaligned. And that is okay.

I asked about the occasional pain I have been experiencing in my back. The answer: nothing in the program should cause that. See a doctor to learn more.

We also talked about my ankle pain. My counselor suggested my running shoes should be replaced with a fresh pair.

Apparently their optimum support status expires after a fairly short duration, six to eight months of use.

That is good to know.

I also was corrected on my thinking about the urinalysis strips that are required in the early days of the program. It turns out that the pink result is not "desired." It is just an indicator of ketosis.

You still can be burning calories when the test strip shows no color. That was another good lesson.

Day: # *100*   Weight: *167.²*

Food & Water

7:00 a.m.	cappuccino		4:45 p.m.	pill (2nd B-12)
8:30 a.m.	pills (1st B-12)		5:00 p.m.	2nd water done
10:00 a.m.	oatmeal, maple		7:00 p.m.	ground beef, lettuce,
10:30 a.m.	1st water done			broccoli, spinach
1:00 p.m.	soup, chicken/rice		7:45 p.m.	cappuccino (decaf)
4:00 p.m.	chocolate bar		8:00 p.m.	3rd water done
6:15 p.m.	chocolate bar			

Exercise

None today.

Comments

It was quite a day. I found myself answering numerous questions about this diet program.

There was an event at work with more than 50 people in attendance.

Many people mentioned that I looked great and whatever I was doing was working well.

On two occasions, I was cornered and interrogated for the diet's particulars.

I was able to provide tons of info and I believe the program may get some new customers.

I am not on the company payroll. I am just a customer and dieter, but I did sound like I was giving a presentation to would-be participants.

I would gain nothing from their decision to partake, but I do believe they would find the program easy and extremely beneficial.

I have obtained an elevated level of happiness and health. And I think it would be great for them to do the same.

Day: #*101*   Weight: *167.*⁴

Food & Water

7:00 a.m.   cappuccino
8:30 a.m.   pills (1st B-12)
10:15 a.m. oatmeal, maple
11:55 a.m. 1st water done
3:00 p.m.   soup, chicken/rice
4:30 p.m.   2nd water done
5:00 p.m.   pills (2nd B-12)

7:00 p.m.   ground chicken,
             broccoli, spinach
7:30 p.m.   cappuccino (decaf)
8:30 p.m.   3rd water done
9:30 p.m.   chocolate bar

Exercise

Weights: bench press, 3 sets; military press, 3 sets; curls (bar), 3 sets; curls (dumbs), 3 sets.

Comments

Today was highly significant in my continual learning of life's lessons.

The potential for a career opportunity presented itself and I had at least a couple of hours of great joy, imagining the situation coming to fruition.

If only I could control my attitude well enough to occupy that mental space at will. That would be a major achievement.

As evidence that such a skill remains beyond my grasp, I submit that there is no real reason for me not to be thinking of that situation in a positive light still.

It is only my mind that has given more weight to the negative aspects—calling it "being realistic"—and settled in to accept that the excellent outcome will not happen.

I am my own enemy in this regard. I need to work harder to channel my thoughts to that realm of great happiness.

Facts are not the true deterrent. The brain creates its own obstacles and it has the power to crush them.

That ability must be harnessed and employed.

Day: #*102*   Weight: *166.*⁶

Food & Water

7:00 a.m.	cappuccino
7:15 a.m.	pills (1st B-12)
9:45 a.m.	oatmeal, maple
10:30 a.m.	1st water done
1:00 p.m.	soup, chicken/rice
1:30 p.m.	pill (2nd B-12)
5:00 p.m.	chocolate bar

5:05 p.m.	2nd water done
7:30 p.m.	talapia, lettuce, broccoli, spinach
8:00 p.m.	cappuccino (decaf)
8:30 p.m.	3rd water done

Exercise

None today.

Comments

There was no announcement over the intercom. No email made the rounds to occupants of the building.

Nevertheless, as I entered our office lounge, I saw a setting that was immediately recognizable.

Two boxes bursting with fresh donuts lay atop a horizontal counter. Out of curiosity, I took a peek.

Yes, all of my old favorites were there. Glazed twisters bumped against chocolate frosted rings and jelly-filled delights.

I closed the lid and commented to a coworker that I was surprised so many of the best flavors had lasted so late in the day.

He remarked that it was the first of the year and everyone's resolutions forbade them from partaking.

"Give it a few weeks," he said. "Then they'll attack a stack of snacks like a school of piranha."

I am glad my diet schedule, and my attitude, have no alignment with the calendar.

I have stuck to my plan and see no obstacle capable of interfering.

Day: #*103*   Weight: *165.*⁶

Food & Water

8:00 a.m.   cappuccino
8:30 a.m.   pills (1st B-12)
9:30 a.m.   1st water done
11:00 a.m.   soup, chicken/rice
11:30 a.m.   2nd water done
2:15 p.m.   oatmeal, maple
4:00 p.m.   3rd water done

5:00 p.m.   chocolate bar
8:00 p.m.   4th water done
8:15 p.m.   pills (2nd B-12)
8:30 p.m.   ground chicken,
             broccoli, spinach,
             lettuce
9:15 p.m.   cappuccino (decaf)

Exercise

Run: 15 minutes w/dog.
Situps: 25.

Comments

I was looking back at my previous entries and noticed my back pain began more than a month ago.

That is a significant period of time. If the suffering had been constant, I most certainly would have consulted a physician before now.

Since it comes and goes and shows no meaningful pattern, I have been able to shrug it off.

But since it has stuck around more than 30 days, I believe I should get it checked out.

It couldn't hurt, right? I know I also need to get a blood test to see how my cholesterol is doing.

It was too high back when I was the beast of blubber.

I am hoping my weight loss and better eating habits of the last three months have remedied that undesirable status.

(My cholesterol) was too high back when I was the beast of blubber.

Day: #*104*   Weight: *165.²*

Food & Water

8:15 a.m.	cappuccino
8:30 a.m.	pills (1st B-12)
10:30 a.m.	1st water done
11:15 a.m.	soup, chicken/rice
11:20 a.m.	2nd water done
2:15 p.m.	chocolate bar
5:15 p.m.	oatmeal, maple

6:30 p.m.	pill (2nd B-12)
7:00 p.m.	ground chicken, broccoli, spinach, lettuce
7:30 p.m.	cappuccino (decaf)
8:00 p.m.	3rd water done

Exercise

None today.

Comments

This morning I was thinking of my energy level and overall condition.

I was comparing my status to an earlier time when, on a self-designed diet and exercise program, I got "in shape" and arrived at the weight I am now.

Back then, however, I was more alert. I could go to bed late and still sit up wide awake two minutes before my alarm was scheduled to sound.

I was full of energy then. I have achieved no similar situation so far in this program.

I believe I know why. My program of the past relied heavily on exercise. My eating was "normal," regular meals without the junk.

My body responded well, dropping the excess fat to get me balanced.

Today's program relies on a reduction in calories to shed the pounds.

I suppose I can hardly expect a high level of energy when my level of nourishment is in a perpetual deficit.

I am certain it all will be right when I reach my goal weight and begin eating my full daily allowance of calories.

Day: #105   Weight: 165.⁰

Food & Water

8:00 a.m.	cappuccino
9:00 a.m.	pills (1st B-12)
9:30 a.m.	1st water done
11:15 a.m.	soup, chicken/rice
11:45 a.m.	2nd water done
2:00 p.m.	chocolate bar
2:45 p.m.	3rd water done

5:00 p.m.	oatmeal, maple
7:00 p.m.	pills (2nd B-12)
7:30 p.m.	yellow fin tuna, broccoli, spinach, lettuce
8:00 p.m.	cappuccino (decaf)

Exercise

Run: 25 minutes w/dog.
Weights: bench press, 3 sets; military press, 3 sets; curls (bar), 3 sets, curls (dumbs), 3 sets.

Comments

I did some research today. I am very interested in the benefits of oatmeal, which I have found to be edible since beginning this diet program.

The oatmeal options on this diet, however, are all "instant" mixes. They are quite different from the whole grain (old fashion) version of oats

It turns out that the instant mix versions contain only half of the fiber and even less percentage of vitamins than the whole oats.

Also, non-program, commercially available instant oatmeal has a considerable amount of sugar.

Apparently, that is not so for the diet plan versions; otherwise there would be difficulty losing weight while eating them.

So, I do plan to try to shift to the whole grain oatmeal after I finish the program. But I also learned that it takes 30 minutes to cook the stovetop version.

Well, I guess that means the more healthful edition will take a bit more effort... much like anything else.

If it is good, you have to work for it.

AFTER FIFTEEN WEEKS

IMPRESSIONS & PROGRESS

A major point of my focus in the past week was my energy level. My diet program counselor always asks about that. Apparently, too much or too little is cause for concern.

I always describe it the same, "neutral." I mean I just feel pretty normal, not great, not bad. I think that is the middle ground they want.

I was remembering when I lost a significant amount of weight on my own through tons of exercise. I lifted a lot of weights. I ran almost every day.

My food intake was ordinary. I ate when hungry. I avoided the junk. I lost massive amounts of fat. I had plenty of energy and felt great.

Nowadays, my energy is more like "blah." That is because this diet is based mostly on taking in fewer calories. It is working. I must be patient. But I am looking forward to increased energy and food intake.

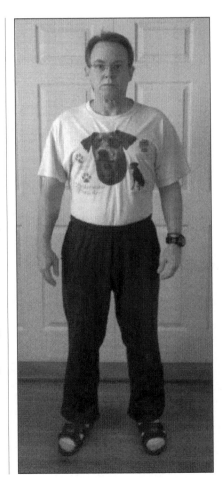

Day: # *106*   Weight: *164.*^{8}

Food & Water

7:00 a.m.	cappuccino
7:30 a.m.	pills (1st B-12)
10:00 a.m.	chocolate bar
11:30 a.m.	1st water done
1:15 p.m.	soup, chicken/rice
4:00 p.m.	oatmeal, maple
4:15 p.m.	2nd water done

4:30 p.m.	pills (2nd B-12)
7:30 p.m.	ground chicken, broccoli, spinach, zucchini
8:00 p.m.	cappuccino (decaf)
8:45 p.m.	3rd water done

Exercise

None today.

Comments

I met with my program counselor today. It was a routine, scheduled visit. All was well with my weight progress.

It was another three-pound week. That is as good as it gets. My blood pressure was just right, too.

We spent a bit of time discussing the various pains I am suffering. She asked if I had gotten new running shoes yet.

That could solve my ankle trouble. She also suggested I have my feet checked to get some inserts that could alleviate my back pain.

Apparently, poor feet

I am willing to give it a try.

alignment within shoes can cause many problems across the body.

I am willing to give it a try. I really need to recover from my maladies as soon as possible.

I am unsure how much longer I can withstand these nagging discomforts.

Day: #*107*   Weight: *164.*⁶

Food & Water

7:30 a.m.	cappuccino
7:35 a.m.	pills (1st B-12)
10:00 a.m.	1st water done
10:30 a.m.	oatmeal, maple
1:30 p.m.	soup, chicken/rice
1:35 p.m.	2nd water done
4:45 p.m.	chocolate bar

7:30 p.m.	cod, broccoli, lettuce, spinach
8:00 p.m.	cappuccino (decaf)
9:00 p.m.	pill (2nd B-12)
9:30 p.m.	3rd water done

Exercise

None today.

Comments

My work caused me to cross paths with an old friend and business associate today.

I had gone without seeing him for several months. It was good to get caught up on his adventures.

About three years ago, he suffered a brutal heart attack. Bypass surgery followed.

He recovered well. He was the epitome of a person with zest for life.

Today, however, he confessed that he was distressed. He regained the 45 pounds he shed to deal with his poor health condition.

It was no surprise, then, that he was extremely interested to hear how I have been so successful in my weight loss efforts.

I explained, of course. I am getting pretty good at presenting the facts of the program.

I think he perked up a bit when I mentioned how easy it is to stay on the plan.

Whichever path he takes to thin, I wish him the best. He is a good guy and the world needs him in it a lot longer.

I will help him, if he asks and I am able.

143

Day: #*108*   Weight: *164.⁰*

Food & Water

7:00 a.m.	cappuccino
9:30 a.m.	pills (1st B-12)
10:00 a.m.	chocolate bar
1:30 p.m.	soup, chicken/rice
1:40 p.m.	1st water done
5:00 p.m.	2nd water done
7:30 p.m.	ground chicken,
	broccoli, spinach, zucchini
8:15 p.m.	cappuccino (decaf)
8:20 p.m.	pill (2nd B-12)
9:30 p.m.	3rd water done
9:40 p.m.	cinnamon bar

Exercise

None today.

Comments

Tonight after dinner, the adults in the family were discussing diets and how some people have difficulty sticking to them or achieving their desired weight.

I noted that I once was in a discussion with a woman about a diet plan that had shown a high rate of success.

She immediately brushed it aside because it prohibited the dieter from eating bread during the program.

That would never work for her, she said, because she "cannot" refrain from that "necessity."

These statements are signs. They are varied as the people who utter them. They all mean the same thing, however.

They indicate the person lacks the ability to try a thing and commit to see it through to a desired outcome.

If you are unwilling to even try to give up bread for a few weeks, you aren't serious about losing weight.

It takes some sacrifice. Bread can return after surplus fat has been chased from the body.

These folks are looking for a program that requires no effort.

That search will come up empty every time.

144

Day: #*109*   Weight: *164.*^{0}

Food & Water

7:00 a.m.	cappuccino
9:45 a.m.	pills (1st B-12)
10:00 a.m.	oatmeal, maple
10:30 a.m.	1st water done
1:15 p.m.	soup, chicken/rice
2:00 p.m.	pill (2nd B-12)
4:00 p.m.	chocolate bar
4:45 p.m.	2nd water done
7:00 p.m.	shrimp, scallops, broccoli, spinach
8:00 p.m.	cappuccino (decaf)
8:30 p.m.	3rd water done

Exercise

Weights: bench press, 3 sets; military press, 3 sets; curls (bar), 3 sets.

Comments

Donuts in the lounge! Again. I am beginning to wonder if all these fat-pill episodes are just my imagination.

I suppose there was proof of their existence today. When I entered the room, a coworker was getting the best of a glazed disk.

I took a peek into the boxes and, despite the late hour, saw two of my old favorites.

There was a jelly-filled, powder-topped donut and a chocolate-covered glazed ring.

I dropped the lid, snickered and headed toward the exit. My coworker seemed astonished and said, "You aren't going to have one?" I said that even a bite would ruin the effort I have invested in my diet.

She said she wished she had the willpower to pass them by, but she was unable to resist.

My thinking is that the trouble she and others experience is an unwillingness to take the first step.

Once you commit and expend some time and money, it is pretty easy to stick with the program.

Day: #*110*   Weight: *163.*²

Food & Water

8:30 a.m.	cappuccino	4:45 p.m.	pill (2nd B-12)
9:15 a.m.	pills (1st B-12)	8:15 p.m.	ground chicken,
11:30 a.m.	oatmeal, maple		spinach, broccoli
11:40 a.m.	1st water done	8:45 p.m.	cappuccino (decaf)
2:00 p.m.	2nd water done	10:15 p.m.	chocolate bar
3:00 p.m.	soup, chicken/rice	10:45 p.m.	4th water done
4:30 p.m.	3rd water done		

Exercise

Run: 20 minutes (w/dog).
Situps: 25 w/kids.

Comments

I enjoyed another pleasant scale reading this morning. It showed me almost a full pound down from yesterday.

I am still thrilled that the weight continues to vanish. I have made no changes. I continue to follow the plan and it keeps working.

I have reached a weight situation where I would expect to have to work harder or take drastic measures to shed the last pounds to arrive at my goal weight.

Of course, I have a substantial amount still to go, but the weight loss is showing no sign of stalling.

It has given me no reason to think it won't continue right down the home stretch to the magic number.

That is reason to be quite happy. I have only about 20 pounds more to shake off.

Compared to the 45 I already have sent packing, that creates no fear of failure.

I am still in control and almost to the finish line. No crowds are roaring for me. No matter, my own satisfaction is all that counts.

I am dieting for selfish reasons. I want good health to maximize my chances for many years in the company of my kids. So, I guess they benefit, too.

Day: #*111*   Weight: *162.*⁸

Food & Water

8:00 a.m.	cappuccino		6:10 p.m.	pill (2nd B-12)
8:15 a.m.	pills (1st B-12)		7:30 p.m.	ahi tuna, broccoli, lettuce
11:00 a.m.	oatmeal, maple		8:00 p.m.	4th water done
11:15 a.m.	1st water done		8:30 p.m.	chocolate bar
2:30 p.m.	2nd water done		9:45 p.m.	cinnamon bar
3:00 p.m.	soup, chicken/rice			
4:00 p.m.	3rd water done			

Exercise

Run: 20 minutes (w/dog).
Weights: squats 3 sets.

Situps: 25.

Comments

When I recently told my program counselor that I was suffering on-and-off back pain, we discussed potential causes.

Eventually, she recommended I get my feet and shoes checked for proper support.

I went to a local retailer and had a computer analyze my stance. It suggested specific inserts for my shoes. I bought them.

When I tried them on at home, they felt great. They provided a good, comfortable lift for my flattened arches.

I stuffed them into my running shoes, leashed the dog and dashed off down the road.

I was feeling good. I added sit-ups and squats. I imagined running more frequently, developing a good, steady habit.

A few hours later, however, my calves were very sore. My back is saying hello, too.

So, I again will try to figure out what is going on with my body.

It is trying to tell me something; that is clear. The exact message remains elusive, though.

147

Day: #*112*   Weight: *162.²*

Food & Water

8:30 a.m.	cappuccino
9:30 a.m.	pills (1st B-12)
11:30 a.m.	oatmeal, maple
12:05 p.m.	1st water done
2:00 p.m.	2nd water done
2:30 p.m.	soup, chicken/rice
7:00 p.m.	cod, broccoli, lettuce,

	spinach
7:30 p.m.	cappuccino (decaf)
7:45 p.m.	pill (2nd B-12)
8:15 p.m.	3rd water done
11:30 p.m.	chocolate bar

Exercise

Run: 20 minutes w/dog.
Weights: bench press, 3 sets; military press, 3 sets; curls (bar), 3 sets.

Comments

Pain continues to interfere with my attempts to function normally. I was feeling okay this morning, so I eagerly jumped into my exercises.

My run tweaked my ankle and reminded me to rethink my approach to aerobic workouts.

I need to exchange the asphalt roadway for the soft conveyer belt of my treadmill.

When lifting weights, curls, actually, I realized what might be stressing my back muscles beyond, or different from, their normal movements.

A little later in the day I was unable to find a position in which to sit or stand that didn't cause me heavy discomfort.

I went to lie on my bed for a while to allow my back to rest. My entire body took advantage.

Even my brain shifted to nap mode and I ended up getting a short amount of sleep. I needed that.

I just wish I could report the incident reduced the trouble my back is giving me, even as I lean over paper to write this (originally by hand in my notebook).

AFTER SIXTEEN WEEKS

IMPRESSIONS & PROGRESS

The most significant event of the last week would have to be a conversation I had with an old friend.

He was feeling a bit down for having regained a lot of weight he previously had dropped in response to a heart attack and subsequent bypass surgery.

He was keen to know more about the program I am pursuing. I told him all I know. I hope he follows through. It is too easy to fall into the old eating traps, to be lured by the scent of pleasurable foods, to devour large quantities of uncounted calories.

I recalled other conversations with overweight friends whose unwillingness to alter their lifestyles is evident in their words. One scoffed at a diet that required obstaining from bread for a time. That "sacrifice" should be a minor footnote to the bigger picture.

Status quo leads us to obesity. We must be willing to change, if we want to be healthy and trim.

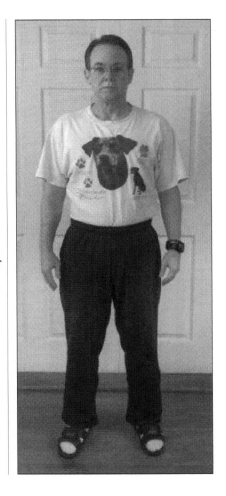

6

Flat spot obtained but not on my belly

*P*lateaus are good, if you are among cliffs and need to pitch a tent. If you are dieting, however, they are welcome as a scorpion in your sleeping bag.

I have no idea why camping metaphors are leaping into my brain. I suppose my mind quickly grabbed something familiar and enjoyable yet easily ruined.

A plateau (period of no weight loss), if not short, can burden the mind, especially when you really need to see some progress.

I guess that time is whenever you are changing your eating schedule with the intent to deprive yourself of a full day's calories.

In the past month, I suffered my most severe stall to date. It lasted seven days. That is a full one-fourth of the period covered in this summary.

Perhaps the stretch of stagnant time was not wasted. Maybe there was something going on I could not see, or understand even if it had shown itself in a way less disguised.

I only know the frustration I felt. I can tell myself repeatedly to focus on the overall program goals and trend of movement forward. Still, I struggled. And I admit I felt helpless.

There is no real action that can be taken to help bust loose from the glitch. You cannot eat fewer calories. That quantity is meticulously measured and must be maintained.

151

Instinct says I could increase the amount of exercise I am doing, but that has limited effect.

Running, for example, burns about 10 calories per minute. That is 600 calories per hour of jaw-jarring, pavement-pounding, body-slamming my way through the neighborhood.

Even if I were to kid myself into thinking I could run a full hour straight, it takes scorching 3,500 calories to result in one pound of fat loss. That would take several days, each with 60 minutes of a physical beating. Not me. Not now. Never.

So, what is a dieter to do? Well, I should know by now. This is not my first flat spell. When it happened before, I talked myself through it.

The experience was rough, sure. But having whipped it, I told myself I had learned enough to sail through the next encounter. I even reminded myself of those lessons while I was battling the big one.

My words of comfort and support failed to conquer my anguish.

I learned another "body and mind" lesson. Throughout my life to this point, awareness of my hunger always seemed to be triggered by something physical, a rumbling of my stomach, a distinct feeling of emptiness in my gut.

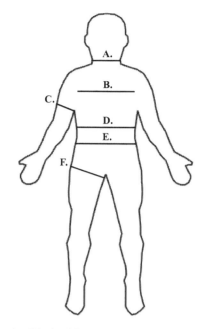

A. Neck: 15

B. Chest: 42

C. Biceps: $12.^5$

D. Waist (navel): 37

E. High Hip (belt line): 35

F. Thighs: $21.^5$

G. Weight: $162.^2$

That seems to be no more.

Nowadays, an alert to my hunger, although slight, arrives in the form of mental images and reminiscing of tastes of excellent (horrible, i.e., high-calorie, high-fat) meals from my past.

152

I have been driving my car when, unprovoked, I would think of shrimp tacos, lobster pasta, eggs Benedict, or some other dastardly heap of calories.

The good thing is that I recognize these visions/thoughts for what they are: a reminder to consume a bit of nutrition.

They are not cravings— although that would be the identification presumed by persons inexperienced in such matters.

A small package of diet-plan soup mixed with water and heated and those dreamy delights disappear from my cranium.

On a final note from the past month, in the continuing saga of "Donuts in the Lounge," fellow employees seemed to be far less interested in the sugary beasts than they have in the past.

It was noted that those good folks are trying to abide by their new year's resolutions.

So, give it a week or two. The devouring will return to a familiar pace.

It still will exclude me, though.

Day: #*113*   Weight: *163.²*

Food & Water

7:00 a.m.	cappuccino		7:00 p.m.	3rd water done
8:00 a.m.	pills (1st B-12)		7:30 p.m.	ahi tuna, lettuce
10:30 a.m.	oatmeal, maple			spinach, broccoli
11:00 a.m.	1st water done		8:00 p.m.	pill (2nd B-12)
1:30 p.m.	soup, chicken/rice		8:30 p.m.	cappuccino (decaf)
1:40 p.m.	2nd water done			
4:20 p.m.	chocolate bar			

Exercise

None today.

Comments

We have so little to talk about these days, my program counselor and me. Obviously, today I had my appointment to get weighed.

I only lost a pound-and-a-half this week, according to their scale. I think mine tells a slightly different story.

Regardless, we didn't have a detailed conversation. I get asked, "What is new?" My answer is, "Nothing." "Do you have any questions?" "No."

She checks my blood pressure. It is fine. I make my food selections and pay. Then, I am on my way.

No news is good news, as they say. The routine is getting streamlined, as it should.

The weight keeps vanishing, albeit slowly.

Nowadays, my desire to get quickly to my goal weight has less to do with wanting to eat regular meals and more to do with being able to shop for clothes that should fit for a while.

This jumping from one size to another is slightly frustrating. I know; all my problems should be so "heavy."

Day: #*114*   Weight: *163.*⁰

Food & Water

7:00 a.m.	cappuccino
8:00 a.m.	pills (1st B-12)
10:00 a.m.	oatmeal, maple
11:05 a.m.	1st water done
1:00 p.m.	soup, chicken/rice
4:00 p.m.	chocolate bar
4:05 p.m.	2nd water done

4:10 p.m.	pill (2nd B-12)
7:00 p.m.	ground chicken, broccoli, lettuce, spinach
7:30 p.m.	cappuccino (decaf)
8:00 p.m.	3rd water done

Exercise

None today.

Comments

Today I had the pleasure of conversing with a fellow employee who went through the same diet program.

We chatted for quite a while about how our lives have changed, how our attitudes toward food and physical conditioning have been altered—for the better—forever.

He noted that he had been large all of his life and the counselors set a goal for him that he achieved on schedule.

He also was proud to add that he exceeded that by five pounds, where his weight remains, the lowest it has been in his adult life.

We talked a lot about foods and how we have no real attraction to the junk anymore.

I admitted that I have a few less-than-perfect meals I want to eat when it is all over.

But I will be much smarter about it, conservative on the amounts, to say the least.

Being smart is the key and we agreed the program has helped us both in that regard.

Day: #*115*   Weight: *163.⁰*

Food & Water

7:15 a.m.	cappuccino
8:30 a.m.	pills (1st B-12)
10:45 a.m.	oatmeal, maple
1:15 p.m.	1st water done
2:45 p.m.	pill (2nd B-12)
3:00 p.m.	soup, chicken/rice
3:15 p.m.	2nd water done

7:00 p.m.	cod, broccoli, spinach, lettuce
7:30 p.m.	cappuccino (decaf)
8:00 p.m.	3rd water done
9:30 p.m.	chocolate bar

Exercise

None today.

Comments

Today, in the course of work, I was drawn into another conversation about dieting.

A long-time coworker was interested to hear the details of the program I am engaging. He is unhappy with his current weight and would like to pursue a program that is certain to succeed.

Seeing my results and learning about the quantity and quality of the foods, he seemed pleased.

I do believe he will go for a free consultation and jump in to this program within a few weeks.

I am hoping I am a step closer to solving the mystery of the source of my back pain. I never considered the current suspect because it wasn't too long ago that we brought it into our home.

I am talking about our bed. I selected the mattress because it was firm. I noticed recently, however, that it seems too squishy.

To test my theory, I am sleeping on the floor for a few days.

If my discomfort subsides, my diet and weight lifting will be cleared of all charges.

Day: #*116* Weight: *163.²*

Food & Water

5:30 a.m.	cappuccino		7:00 p.m.	3rd water done
9:20 a.m.	pills (1st B-12)		7:15 p.m.	ground chicken, broccoli, lettuce, spinach
9:30 a.m.	oatmeal, maple			
1:30 p.m.	1st water done			
2:15 p.m.	soup, chicken/rice		7:45 p.m.	pill (2nd B-12)
4:30 p.m.	2nd water done		8:00 p.m.	cappuccino (decaf)
5:00 p.m.	chocolate bar			

Exercise

None today.

Comments

I suppose if I were going to have trouble on this diet, it would have shown itself today.

We had our company's annual all-employee breakfast. I am part of the setup team, so I worked through the entire event.

I also never have been much of a breakfast eater. So, the potential for difficulty came later when the caterer's leftovers were brought back to the office building and spread out for all to enjoy in the employee lounge.

I walked in and immediately spotted a 24-inch-long tray packed full of French toast slices.

I mentioned to a coworker that, if I were still eating according to my old ways, I could put a major dent in that quantity.

She asked why I wasn't partaking at all and I explained that I was dieting. She said, "Why, doctor's orders?" I said the orders were mine.

I needed/wanted to lose weight for numerous reasons. It was an odd exchange. And I left without touching the offerings.

But I did reminisce about how much I enjoyed that selection at a previous point in my life.

157

Day: #*117*   Weight: *161.*⁴

Food & Water

8:30 a.m.	cappuccino	5:55 p.m.	chocolate bar
8:45 a.m.	pills (1st B-12)	8:30 p.m.	shrimp, broccoli,
10:45 a.m.	oatmeal, maple		spinach, lettuce
11:30 a.m.	1st water done	8:00 p.m.	pill (2nd B-12)
2:00 p.m.	2nd water done	9:00 p.m.	3rd water done
3:30 p.m.	soup, chicken/rice	9:30 p.m.	cappuccino (decaf)
4:00 p.m.	3rd water done		

Exercise

Run: 20 minutes w/dog.
Situps: 25

Comments

Last night I dreamed I was on a diet. No real surprise there, right? My friends knew I was dieting, so, when they saw me, they brought lunch for all of us. For me, that meant a cheeseburger with a lettuce wrapping.

Many of the fast-food chains offer a sandwich like that. Well, of course, that is prohibited in my program.

It wasn't reality, though. So, refusing their kind offer was no problem. There were no hurt feelings.

The dream has me puzzled, however. I am wondering whether my mind fed me that scenario because I am still very conscious of my diet and a substantial amount of time still lies ahead.

Or, was it because I have been on the program so long that it has become a part of my life?

And, maybe it is both.

I guess it has no real relevance whatever the answer.

But the mind is a major player in this journey and it needs to be cared for in a way that makes it a partner rather than a foe—or even a mere observer.

Day: #*118*   Weight: *161.*^{0}

Food & Water

9:00 a.m.	oatmeal, maple
9:05 a.m.	pills (1st B-12)
12:10 p.m.	1st water done
12:30 p.m.	soup, chicken/rice
3:25 p.m.	2nd water done
4:00 p.m.	soup, beef/veggie
5:30 p.m.	3rd water done

7:00 p.m.	ground pork, spinach broccoli, lettuce,
7:30 p.m.	pill (2nd B-12)
7:40 p.m.	cappuccino (decaf)
8:45 p.m.	4th water done
9:15 p.m.	chocolate pudding

Exercise

Run: 20 minutes w/dog.
Weights: bench press, 3 sets; military press, 3 sets; curls (bar), 3 sets; curls (dumbs), 3 sets.

Comments

My wife, she may be on to something. I mentioned to her this morning that I had dreamed again about being back in the Navy.

This one was different from so many I have had in recent years.

In those, the good experience always was destroyed by a discovery that my uniform was unmistakenly wrong. These were no small malfunctions. Many times I found myself wearing the wrong-color shirt. Frequently, I was wearing a rank that was below the level I actually achieved.

Since I have such fond memories of my time in the service, dreaming about that came as no surprise. The uniform problems, however, were a significant puzzle.

I thought the uniform issue represented unfinished business with the military. My wife offered another perspective.

She said the blemished dreams may have been my mind telling me my body was wrong (overweight) and needed fixing.

Since I have made major improvements in that regard, and the dreams are continuing without the uniform discrepancies, that may have been the exact cause.

I hope so.

Day: #*119*   Weight: *161.⁰*

Food & Water

8:00 a.m.	cappuccino	7:15 p.m.	cod, broccoli,
9:00 a.m.	pills (1st B-12)		spinach, lettuce
11:00 a.m.	oatmeal, maple	7:30 p.m.	3rd water done
11:15 a.m.	1st water done	7:45 p.m.	cappuccino (decaf)
2:00 p.m.	chocolate bar	9:30 p.m.	pill (2nd B-12)
2:45 p.m.	2nd water done	10:00 p.m.	4th water done
5:30 p.m.	cinnamon crunch bar		

Exercise

Situps: 25.

Comments

I spent a fair amount of time today researching oatmeal. I am not obsessed. And I do have a life.

I just believe the health benefits connected to that meal make it worth adding to my daily routine.

Unfortunately, I am unable to eat that just yet. But I am so eager to try out the whole grain variety that my mind has been hovering on it.

The only action available to me concerning oatmeal was to learn as much as I can about the different options.

I have heard about the "old fashioned" type and the "steel cut" version.

In the store today, I also saw a "quick-cooking" edition. The quick oats should not be confused with "instant" oatmeal. The quick type is offered for old fashioned (whole) and steel cut (chopped).

All three have nearly identical vitamins, fiber, etc. The old fashioned is said to be crunchy. The steel cut is reportedly creamier. The quick oats just take less time to cook.

I will take the fast, creamy oatmeal for smoothness and health, thanks.

Total pounds lost so far: 46.⁰

**Total pounds
lost so far:
46.^{0}**

AFTER SEVENTEEN WEEKS

IMPRESSIONS & PROGRESS

This past week was marked by a couple of dreams.

They were notable because they seemed to deal with my diet pursuits and puzzled me about my subconscious mind.

I dreamed of ordering at a fast-food establishment, but I got a burger wrapped in lettuce instead of a bread bun.

Of course, such a meal has no place in this portion of my program. It is interesting to see, however, the thinking that arrives in my sleep.

Another dream involved my past in the Navy. I have had such dreams over the years, but this one showed no "uniform" problems.

It was suggested that wearing the wrong shirt, etc., symbolized something wrong that needed to be corrected, my overweight body, for example.

This problem-free dream could mean my subconscious mind is acknowledging the diet success I have achieved thus far.

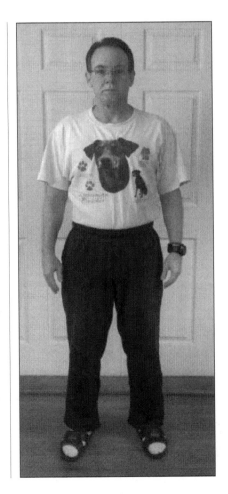

Day: #*120*   Weight: *160.*⁴

Food & Water

7:15 a.m.   cappuccino
7:45 a.m.   pills (1st B-12)
10:30 a.m.   oatmeal, maple
10:45 a.m.   1st water done
1:45 p.m.   soup, chicken/rice
1:50 p.m.   2nd water done
4:15 p.m.   chocolate bar

5:00 p.m.   pill (2nd B-12)
7:00 p.m.   ground chicken,
             broccoli, spinach,
             lettuce
7:30 p.m.   cappuccino (decaf)
8:00 p.m.   3rd water done

Exercise

None today.

Comments

I met with my program counselor today. I got the full computerized analysis. Unfortunately, I got some bad news.

I lost 10 pounds since the last time I got a complete inspection. While that sounds good, more than half of the weight I lost was muscle.

To me, that is tragic.

I have been working hard to build muscle. Instead, I get the reversal.

My counselor said to increase the size of my protein portion of my "normal" meal. This I will do gladly. It means a little more food to fill me.

Another interesting thing happened. They are running a "special." If I were to purchase an extra box of meals (seven day supply), my name would be entered into a raffle. The winner will get a week of free meals.

I gave it a moment of thought. I didn't like the odds. They were heavily against me.

I understand they are running a business. And everybody likes a shot at getting something for nothing. A week of free food would be awesome, there's no doubt about that, but I passed.

I need no extra.

Day: #*121*   Weight: *160.⁶*

Food & Water

7:10 a.m.	cappuccino
7:35 a.m.	pills (1st B-12)
10:30 a.m.	oatmeal, maple
1:45 p.m.	soup, chicken/rice
2:30 p.m.	1st water done
4:05 p.m.	chocolate bar
4:10 p.m.	pill (2nd B-12)

4:30 p.m.	2nd water done
7:00 p.m.	talapia, zucchini, lettuce
7:30 p.m.	cappuccino (decaf)
8:00 p.m.	3rd water done

Exercise

Weights: bench press, 3 sets; curls (dumbs), 3 sets.

Sit-ups: 25.

Comments

I finally saw a doctor today about my back pain. There were no obvious answers. He had no suspicion about my diet or things I was missing.

So, blood was taken. Tests will be performed.

The pain is centered where my kidneys reside. So, that is the focus of the investigation.

I also will be getting some physical therapy to deal with any muscle-related issues.

I am looking forward to an end to this discomfort.

I had another coworker inquire about this program today. It was interesting comparing our bad eating habits.

Mine have changed, of course. I hope he decides to engage and enjoy the quick and relatively easy weight loss.

He is a good guy and I would like to see him happy and healthy very soon.

Since I suffered muscle loss recently, I was told to add some more protein across the board, even if I am not exercising that day.

Tonight I ate 10 ounces of talapia. It was quite filling.

Day: #*122*   Weight: *159.*⁸

Food & Water

7:10 a.m.	cappuccino		7:00 p.m.	ground chicken, broccoli, lettuce
7:30 a.m.	pills (1st B-12)		7:30 p.m.	peanut butter bar
12:30 p.m.	oatmeal, maple		8:00 p.m.	3rd water done
1:00 p.m.	1st water done		9:00 p.m.	chocolate bar
4:20 p.m.	soup, chicken/rice			
4:30 p.m.	2nd water done			
4:45 p.m.	pill (2nd B-12)			

Exercise

None today.

Comments

Today was a pretty big test. My workplace is almost famous for the frequency that food is presented.

Lunch today was a potluck affair worthy of note. I brought salad, even though I would be eating none of the selections.

As I sat near the television, a coworker asked if my diet program permitted me to take a day off. Could I eat wildly and resume the schedule tomorrow?

I said I had never discussed the issue with my counselor because the thought never entered my head until he asked. I mentioned that any bites not in my lineup would waste my entire day's efforts and I found that unacceptable.

I am trying to achieve my goal weight in the shortest time possible while remaining healthy.

That only can be accomplished by sticking to the plan. He said he understood.

Another coworker noticed I was able to ignore all the fantastic soups and array of cakes, cookies, brownies and other desserts.

She complimented me on my willpower. I said that I was on autopilot. My routine made it easy to resist that stuff.

Day: #*123*   Weight: *159.*^{8}

Food & Water

7:00 a.m.	cappuccino
7:45 a.m.	pills (1st B-12)
9:30 a.m.	1st water done
10:20 a.m.	oatmeal, maple
1:30 p.m.	soup, chicken/rice
2:30 p.m.	2nd water done
6:00 p.m.	peanut butter bar
4:30 p.m.	2nd water done
7:00 p.m.	talapia, broccoli, lettuce
8:30 p.m.	3rd water done
10:30 p.m.	peanut butter bar

Exercise

Sit-ups: 25.
Squats, 3 sets.

Comments

When I began this program, one of the first things that seemed like work was having to write down all of my activities, eating, drinking, taking pills.

Those are still tasks, but today I realized that all that time etching my actions onto paper has served me pretty well.

I discovered that I was hitting the time marks just from habit. The light bulb went off in my head and told me that I can continue on these good habits after the diet is over—without having to think too much about it.

It all has become second nature. I am unsure whether that was a main reason for requiring written entries in a log book. If not, it certainly seems to be a beneficial by-product.

If I nagged about it before... well... never mind.

...etching my actions onto paper has served me pretty well.

Day: #*124*   Weight: *159.*⁴

Food & Water

8:30 a.m.	oatmeal, maple	6:15 p.m.	peanut butter bar
9:00 a.m.	pills (1st B-12)	6:30 p.m.	pill (2nd B-12)
11:00 a.m.	1st water done	8:30 p.m.	ground chicken, lettuce, broccoli
11:45 a.m.	soup, chicken/rice		
12:05 p.m.	2nd water done	9:30 p.m.	4th water done
3:15 p.m.	chili, beef/veggie	10:00 p.m.	cinnamon crunch bar
4:30 p.m.	3rd water done		

Exercise

Run: 20 minutes w/dog.
Weights: bench press, 3 sets; military press, 3 sets; curls (bar), 3 sets; curls (bells) 3 sets.

Comments

I worked out like a beast today. I could feel my weight-lifting was having more effect than usual.

I worked the same weight, but I lifted faster and allowed less time to pass between sets.

The immediate onset of soreness was an indication of a successful event. My run was good, too.

I really knew at the end of my usual distance because I kept going for a bit more and still felt good.

I remembered back in the chubby days being exhausted and thrilled to reach the designated finish line.

The lighter I get, the easier the run becomes.

Papers came in the mail today from the doctor's office.

They were supposed to provide details of my recent examination to determine the cause of my back pain.

There were three pages. They were marked "1 of 4," "2 of 4," and "3 of 4."

I suppose the info I needed was on page 4, wherever that went. Thanks, doc!

Day: #*125*   Weight: *159.*⁴

Food & Water

9:15 a.m.   cappuccino
10:00 a.m. pills (1st B-12)
12:30 p.m. soup, chicken/rice
12:45 p.m. 1st water done
2:30 p.m.   2nd water done
3:30 p.m.   chocolate pudding
3:45 p.m.   3rd water done

7:30 p.m.   salmon, lettuce,
            broccoli
7:45 p.m.   4th water done
8:00 p.m.   cappuccino (decaf)
8:25 p.m.   pill (2nd B-12)
9:00 p.m.   chocolate bar

Exercise

Run: 20 minutes w/dog.
Sit-ups: 25.

Weights: squats, 3 sets.

Comments

We made the rounds through all the major aisles at Costco today.

If you have no Costco or never shopped at one, it is a great place to get groceries. They have excellent prices for buying in larger quantities.

I note the place here because it has another characteristic for which it is famous.

There are numerous cooked or mixed food samples that are free for the taking. And that is a situation of concern to a dieter.

Temptation lurks at every turn. My wife and kids and their grandmother enjoyed several tasty morsels. Me, I just pushed the cart and thought about the diet plan soup that was waiting for me at home.

It really was easy to pass by those offerings. I continue to find pleasure in possessing that ability.

But, make no mistake. I am getting near the end of my trip. I am almost at my goal weight.

When I move off of the diet, I will gladly have some bites of my old favorites—only in moderation, of course.

Day: #*126*   Weight: *159.*^{*0*}

Food & Water

7:00 a.m.	cappuccino	4:30 p.m.	pill (2nd B-12)
7:30 a.m.	pills (1st B-12)	7:30 p.m.	scallops, shrimp,
10:10 a.m.	oatmeal, maple		lettuce, broccoli,
11:20 a.m.	1st water done		zucchini
1:15 p.m.	soup, chicken/rice	8:00 p.m.	3rd water done
1:30 p.m.	2nd water done	9:00 p.m.	chocolate pudding
4:15 p.m.	chocolate bar		

Exercise

Weights: bench press, 3 sets; curls (bar), 3 sets; curls (dumbs) 3 sets.

Comments

It has been a day of some confusion. I got some papers in the mail from my doctor. I had gone to get my kidneys checked.

My back was hurting and I wanted to confirm my diet was not stressing those organs.

Well, the papers told me nothing. I had thought a page was missing. Maybe there was.

I called the doctor's office to get a clear answer. They said my kidneys were functioning normally.

That is a relief. So, by process of elimination, I must have strained the muscles.

I deliberated and decided my method of doing curls with a bar was over-taxing my back.

So, eager to remedy that, I adjusted and hit the weights.

The altered curl positioning confirmed that my back had been assisting. Tonight's curls hurt the arms a lot more. I really felt the biceps cry a little. Good workout.

One problem: my back is hurting again. Same spot.

To top off the weird day, the mail contained my blood test results, confirming my kidneys are probably my best feature at the moment.

18

**Total pounds
lost so far:
48.^{0}**

AFTER EIGHTEEN WEEKS

IMPRESSIONS & PROGRESS

No rest for the ambitious! A coworker asked if my diet program allowed me to take a "day off" and ignore the calorie, fat and carbohydrate levels of the food consumed and then get "back on track" the following day.

I suppose then the dieter would act like it never happened.

I explained that a benefit—and necessary element—of my diet is the development of new attitudes and habits.

So, I had (have) no desire to "binge" eat. That is because I want no delay achieving my goal.

The episode also highlighted the difference between me and people who are not engaged in fat reduction pursuits: our thinking.

I believe no significant weight reduction will occur for anyone who is looking for a vacation from sensible eating.

True, lasting change requires commitment, an attitude alteration. I am happy I have embraced it.

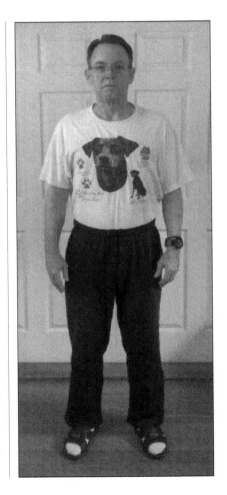

169

Day: #*127*   Weight: *159.*⁴

Food & Water

7:15 a.m.   oatmeal, maple
7:40 a.m.   pills (1st B-12)
11:30 a.m. soup, chicken/rice
12:05 p.m. 1st water done
4:00 p.m.   2nd water done
4:15 p.m.   peanut butter bar
4:20 p.m.   pill (2nd B-12)

7:30 p.m.   ground chicken,
            lettuce, broccoli,
            spinach
8:00 p.m.   3rd water done
10:15 p.m. cinnamon crunch bar

Exercise

None today.

Comments

My day began with a bit of frustration. A jump onto the scale showed my weight up four-tenths of a pound from yesterday.

I have experienced such rises enough by now that I don't get too riled. But this seemed to be associated with a recent across-the-board increase in the protein portion of my "normal" meal.

So, it got me to thinking. If my weight drop hits a snag and stalls, at what point do I quit this program and shift into my own program?

There is at least one advantage to following through on that. If I return to regular, smart eating or a full day's calories, I will have increased energy.

That would enable me to workout much harder and burn the remaining unwanted fat. I remember fondly my workout schedule and energy level of the past.

I thought I might at least hint of my possible plan when I met my program counselor later in the morning. But her scale showed I had dropped two pounds for the week. All is normal.

Never mind!

Day: #*128*   Weight: *158.*⁸

Food & Water

7:15 a.m.	oatmeal, maple		10:00 p.m.	salmon, lettuce, broccoli, zucchini, spinach
8:00 a.m.	pills (1st B-12)			
9:10 a.m.	1st water done		10:10 p.m.	3rd water done
10:20 a.m.	soup, chicken/rice		10:15 p.m.	pill (2nd B-12)
1:10 p.m.	sloppy joe		10:30 p.m.	chocolate chip cookie
3:30 p.m.	2nd water done			
4:15 p.m.	peanut butter bar			

Exercise

Run: 25 minutes w/dog.
Weights: bench press, 4 sets.

Comments

I have been giving some thought to the number of meals I eat in a day.

It works very well while dieting and consuming a reduced amount of calories.

I eat frequently enough that I never really get hungry. That is good. But I am a bit concerned that I am training my body to expect this arrangement to continue long-term.

I do not imagine that I will be eating so many times in a day when I return to "normal" eating.

Maybe my program counselor will advise me to continue at this frequency of meals after transitioning off of the diet.

I suppose I could do that, but I will have to learn what items could be filling and yet not put me over my daily calorie limit.

That is accomplished now by eating diet-plan packaged meals. I guarantee I will not continue to buy those things in the distant future.

No matter how good many of them taste, that routine must end.

171

Day: #*129* Weight: *159.*⁰

Food & Water

7:00 a.m.	oatmeal, maple
8:00 a.m.	pills (1st B-12)
10:00 a.m.	1st water done
10:30 a.m.	sloppy joe
10:35 a.m.	2nd water done
1:30 p.m.	soup, chicken/rice
1:45 p.m.	3rd water done

4:30 p.m.	peanut butter bar
7:45 p.m.	beef, broccoli, lettuce
8:15 p.m.	4th water done
8:30 p.m.	pill (2nd B-12)
9:15 p.m.	chocolate chip cookie

Exercise

Sit-ups: 25.
Run: 20 minutes w/dog.

Weights: squats, 3 sets.

Comments

I had a Rocky Balboa moment today. One of my motivators to lose a lot of weight was a photo of me skateboarding when I was a teenager. I was very lean.

Back then, I felt I needed to put on weight. The reality was that I looked pretty good.

I was fit. I stared at the photo and asked myself why I couldn't look like that again. I convinced myself that only a large amount of body fat stood between me and that figure.

So, I launched into this diet program. As my physique sheds the blubber, my outline is moving closer to match that skinny kid of my early days.

But, then, today, that Rocky thing happened. In the film, the brawler sat up in his bed and admitted he had no chance to whip the champ.

He realized his goal needed to be "going the distance" with his opponent.

For me, my well-aged skin and bones are proof I never again will look like my younger self.

And that is okay. I will settle happily for looking like a geezer in great shape and excellent health.

Day: #*130*   Weight: *158.*^{0}

Food & Water

7:15 a.m.	cappuccino
8:30 a.m.	pills (1st B-12)
10:45 a.m.	oatmeal, maple
11:00 a.m.	1st water done
1:30 p.m.	soup, chicken/rice
2:45 p.m.	2nd water done
4:30 p.m.	pill (2nd B-12)

7:30 p.m.	ground chicken, broccoli, zucchini, spinach
8:00 p.m.	3rd water done
9:30 p.m.	chocolate chip cookie

Exercise

None today.

Comments

Today I felt like I was more mentally alert than usual.

Maybe I should describe it, rather, as being a bit more enthused to take on tasks.

I grabbed a package and some papers and bolted away from work at lunch time.

Usually, I am content to sit in the lounge and catch some news on the television.

Instead, I had a good feeling about being out and about and delivering to a shipping company and our kids' school district offices.

I am unsure where my enthusiasm originated. It may have begun in the early morning when I found I weighed a pound less than yesterday.

That frequently helps me to feel uplifted. And I should not make too much of it.

I expect I will have many more days of such "readiness to do" since I have a great feeling of satisfaction from having gotten my weight back in control and my body into better shape.

173

Day: #*131*   Weight: *157.*⁶

Food & Water

8:45 a.m.	oatmeal, maple	7:30 p.m.	chocolate bar
9:00 a.m.	pills (1st B-12)	9:00 p.m.	ground chicken,
11:30 a.m.	1st water done		broccoli, lettuce,
1:25 a.m.	2nd water done		spinach
1:35 p.m.	soup, chicken/rice	9:30 p.m.	4th water done
4:15 p.m.	3rd water done	10:00 p.m.	pill (2nd B-12)
4:30 p.m.	chocolate bar	10:15 p.m.	chocolate chip cookie

Exercise

Run: 20 minutes (w/dog).
Weights: bench press (wide), 3 sets; benchS (narrow), 3 sets; curls (bar) 3, sets; curls (dumbs), 3 sets.

Comments

I found myself staring across the kitchen this morning. My eyes locked onto a batch of firm-looking bananas on a counter top.

Of course, I am unable to devour one on this diet program. Peeking into my future, though, I could imagine enjoying that great-tasting and filling nutritional snack.

Somehow, that thought led me to a question: how will I keep myself motivated to munch a banana instead of a burrito when I have complete freedom of choice?

My initial response is that I need physical fitness goals, such as triathlons or bodybuilding competitions.

Admittedly, one of those seems pretty far fetched. I already have competed, however, in an Olympic-distance triathlon.

If I were to set my sights on bodybuilding, I could approach it in similar fashion.

I acknowledged to myself that my intention was not to win. It was just to be involved and benefit from the training.

Obviously, these ideas need some more thought to create a plan. But I have taken the first step!

Day: #*132*   Weight: *158.*⁴

Food & Water

8:30 a.m.   cappuccino
9:15 a.m.   pills (1st B-12)
11:30 a.m. oatmeal, maple
11:40 a.m. 1st water done
2:15 p.m.   chocolate bar
5:30 p.m.   2nd water done
7:30 p.m.   talapia, spinach,

          broccoli
8:00 p.m.   3rd water done
9:00 p.m.   pill (2nd B-12)
9:15 p.m.   chocolate chip cookie
10:45 p.m. chocolate bar

Exercise

Run: 20 minutes w/dog.
Run: 10 minutes on treadmill.

Comments

Well, I thought I had my back problem close to being nailed down.

Then, I go through most all of today without problem until early evening. I lifted no weights today. I did no sit-ups.

So, I should have suffered no back pain today. Wrong!

While sitting at my desk and typing, the discomfort became almost unbearable.

I fidget around looking for a painless position and am unable to find one. So, back to the mystery.

Is it my posture? It is the same one I have used for many years without trouble.

Could it be that my run through the neighborhood is affecting my back? There is timing there that could suggest a connection.

I hate to stop that for several days just to see if the pain leaves town.

I guess I could go back to swimming for a while. I have been wanting to do that, anyway.

So, I will give it a try and see what happens. More info to come.

Day: #*133* Weight: *157.*⁶

Food & Water

9:30 a.m.	cappuccino	9:30 p.m.	beef, cauliflower, broccoli
11:20 a.m.	oatmeal, maple	8:00 p.m.	3rd water done
11:30 a.m.	pills (1st B-12)	9:30 p.m.	chocolate chip cookie
11:40 a.m.	1st water done	9:40 p.m.	pill (2nd B-12)
2:30 p.m.	chocolate bar		
6:15 p.m.	cinnamon crunch bar		
6:30 p.m.	2nd water done		

Exercise

None today.

Comments

Okay, the back pain saga continues. A little light may have been shed on the situation, however.

I wrote a note to myself this morning. It was a reminder that I was not experiencing any discomfort in my back. I suppose that could be said for most of the day.

I remember telling my doctor that the pain came and went seemingly at random because I had been unable to see a pattern.

As I write this, I am in a bad way. My back is hurting. It began an hour or so ago. I was sitting at my computer desk when the pain began. I will not blame my chair, though. It could be posture, but I doubt that.

It might be the result of a day on my feet. But why now? So, in my weight-loss adventure, did I lose back muscle? That could explain it.

If that is the case, it may take me a while to build that up again. I suppose I shall research to learn the likelihood that weakness is the culprit.

Then I must figure what the best exercise is to remedy the issue.

AFTER NINETEEN WEEKS

IMPRESSIONS & PROGRESS

Repetition is conditioning. It creates habits. It permits expectations.

I am getting comfortable eating six times each day. There is much to like about this routine.

I am never hungry and I never eat so much that I feel bloated or weighted down. Without those issues, there also is no guilt.

So, the benefits seem obvious. But the schedule makes me wonder how it will be converted to post-diet life.

Will I continue this frequency of feeding my body? If so, will the portions change as the foods change? If not, will the quantity be altered to counter the number of meals?

There must be some significant adjustment coming because food selections eventually will exclude the packages sold by the diet company and my calorie intake will climb to "normal" levels.

I am eager to get the answers.

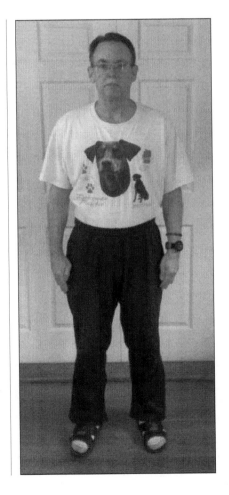

Day: #*134*   Weight: *157.*⁶

Food & Water

7:00 a.m.	cappuccino	4:55 p.m.	cinnamon crunch bar
8:30 a.m.	pills (1st B-12)	7:30 p.m.	ground chicken,
10:30 a.m.	oatmeal, maple		broccoli, lettuce,
11:45 a.m.	1st water done		cauliflower
2:00 p.m.	soup, chicken/rice	8:00 p.m.	pill (2nd B-12)
3:15 p.m.	2nd water done	8:10 p.m.	4th water done
4:45 p.m.	3rd water done	9:45 p.m.	chocolate chip cookie

Exercise

None today.

Comments

At today's Why Weight? appointment, my counselor and I had an interesting discussion.

She asked if I drink diet sodas. I noted that I had stayed away from them completely for about the first four months of my program.

Lately, however, I have been drinking them on occasion, especially when I want a cold drink to go with my hot soup for lunch.

She mentioned that most diet drinks today are sweetened with Aspartame.

She said it is a synthetic material and the body doesn't always know how to deal with it. Sometimes, the body will eject it. Other times it will hang on to it.

For people in the latter category, it can actually cause them to gain body fat.

That is no good for anyone, especially dieters.

So, I will be researching to find some diet drinks that use a better method of mimicking the flavor of sugar.

Day: #*135*   Weight: *157.^{0}*

Food & Water

7:00 a.m.	oatmeal, blueberry		5:05 p.m.	pill (2nd B-12)
8:00 a.m.	pills (1st B-12)		7:45 p.m.	ground chicken, broccoli, lettuce, spinach
8:40 a.m.	1st water done			
11:00 a.m.	soup, crab			
1:05 p.m.	2nd water done		8:15 p.m.	3rd water done
2:00 p.m.	soup, chicken/rice		9:40 p.m.	chocolate chip cookie
5:00 p.m.	chocolate bar			

Exercise

None today.

Comments

Today I introduced a couple of new food items into my lineup. I also dropped one.

I have begun most days with a mug of cappuccino. I have been wanting to move away from that, though.

I like it too much and figure that, if I don't ease off now, it will be more difficult later.

So, I began the day with oatmeal. This one, however, was blueberry.

It was my first time. I must say I enjoyed it.

Interestingly, the smell is strong. The taste is much weaker.

It is good. I am just wondering how to punch up the flavor a bit.

I followed that oatmeal with another first for me, crab soup. Now that flavor was pretty hearty.

I still added a little spice. But it probably needed none.

My third meal was chicken and rice soup, a favorite.

After those meals, I felt like I was sufficiently filled. So, I didn't feel slighted when my fourth meal was a little chocolate bar.

It was a very satisfying day of eating.

Day: #*136*   Weight: *157.*⁴

Food & Water

7:30 a.m.	oatmeal, maple	4:30 p.m.	soup, chicken/rice
8:05 a.m.	pills (1st B-12)	7:30 p.m.	salmon, broccoli,
10:15 a.m.	1st water done		lettuce, spinach
10:30 a.m.	soup, crab	8:00 p.m.	3rd water done
1:00 p.m.	chocolate bar	9:30 p.m.	chocolate bar
3:30 p.m.	2nd water done		
4:10 p.m.	pill (2nd B-12)		

Exercise

None today.

Comments

Well, all it took was another uptick in my weight this morning to get me thinking again about quitting this diet program.

I guess this thinking is aided by my counselor's note that calorie burning frequently slows when a person gets much lighter, as I have done.

This makes me want to know how body builders take off the last few pounds of body fat just before a competition.

I don't believe they stretch that out over several weeks. So, maybe that method would serve me better.

I will research it.

Well, that is my plan.

I have mentioned the idea before and was lulled back to complacency by a return to calorie burning and a favorable reading from my scale.

I must admit. That could happen again. It is no problem, if I am showing progress.

The method is less important than the result.

180

Day: # *137*   Weight: *156.*⁸

Day: # **137**   Weight: **156.**^8

Food & Water

7:15 a.m.	oatmeal, blueberry
8:00 a.m.	pills (1st B-12)
9:45 a.m.	1st water done
10:30 a.m.	soup, crab
1:30 p.m.	soup, chicken/rice
4:30 p.m.	oatmeal, maple
4:40 p.m.	2nd water done

4:45 p.m.	pill (2nd B-12)
8:00 p.m.	lobster, talapia, broccoli, lettuce, spinach
8:15 p.m.	3rd water done
10:45 p.m.	chocolate bar

Exercise

None today.

Comments

As I suspected, a slight drop in my weight this morning pretty much erased my thoughts about dropping this diet program in exchange for some other methods of burning the last of my body fat.

But my amnesia may last as little as a day, depending what the scale tells me tomorrow.

I was sitting at my desk at work and, for some unknown reason, I looked down toward my stomach.

I saw a roll in my shirt. I grabbed at it. I clutched a hunk of fat.

"Hey," I thought, "that's not supposed to be there."

It was a reminder that I have more work to do. No argument. By all acccounts, however, my current condition is very normal.

My coworkers are in disbelief that I am still dieting. So, I want to be sure I am not going too far.

I know the medical charts say I am still overweight. But I don't want to obsess about it.

That would be mentally unhealthy.

So, I must remember to keep my ambition in check.

181

Day: #*138*   Weight: *156.⁰*

Food & Water

8:30 a.m.	oatmeal, blueberry	6:00 p.m.	4th water done
9:00 a.m.	pills (1st B-12)	8:00 p.m.	ground chicken,
9:45 a.m.	1st water done		broccoli, lettuce,
11:15 a.m.	2nd water done		spinach
11:30 a.m.	chocolate bar	9:05 p.m.	pill (2nd B-12)
3:30 p.m.	soup, crab	9:15 p.m.	chocolate chip cookie
4:15 p.m.	3rd water done	11:45 p.m.	chocolate bar

Exercise

Run: 25 minutes (w/dog), 30 minutes on treadmill.

Weights: bench press, 4 sets; curls (bar), 3 sets; curls (dumbs), 3 sets.

Comments

I had an excellent workout today.

I haven't done any real exercise in a few days, trying to heal my ailments.

When I hit it today, I was fresh and it felt great.

My dog and I did our regular route through our neighborhood.

When I got back to the house, I leaped onto my treadmill, turned up my music and did an additional 30 minutes.

By then, I was cooking. I worked the barbells with my upper body muscles.

It was a great strain. I knew I was working it well.

Another indication that it was a highly effective outing are my muscles singing a song of soreness as I move my pen across the paper to make this entry in my log.

It is not a crushing pain. It is merely a reminder that the method works to build muscle.

First the muscle fibers get torn under stress. Then they heal stronger and larger.

And so the cycle continues.

Day: #*139*   Weight: *155.*²

Food & Water

8:45 a.m.	oatmeal, maple
9:15 a.m.	pills (1st B-12)
10:15 a.m.	1st water done
12:15 p.m.	soup, crab
12:45 p.m.	2nd water done
3:00 p.m.	chocolate bar
7:00 p.m.	pill (2nd B-12)

7:30 p.m.	ground chicken, broccoli, lettuce, cauliflower, zucchini
8:30 p.m.	3rd water done
9:30 p.m.	chocolate chip cookie
10:30 p.m.	chocolate bar

Exercise

Run: 25 minutes (w/dog). Weights: squats, 3 sets; calf raises, 3 sets. Lower abs: bridges, 2 sets; leg lifts, 2 sets.

Comments

While I was running today, I thought again about my energy level, comparing it to years ago when I got down to this weight.

Admittedly, my energy level is lower now today because I take in fewer calories to lose fat through diet rather than almost all by exercise.

I remembered that back then I ran an Olympic-distance triathlon. That was about a kilometer swim, 25-mile bike ride and six-mile run.

Today my short run through the neighborhood was enough punishment to make me think the idea of a more challenging race was ludicrous.

I do want to pick some races to use as workout goals, though. This tells me it will be a while before I can even think about that.

I went shopping today at an outlet mall and stocked up on some new shirts... smaller shirts.

These are the size and type that will constantly remind me that I am thinner and prohibit me from putting on any poundage, lest I notice the growth instantly.

I need such an indicator because I never want to be big again.

I like the new me.

Day: #*140*   Weight: *156.*⁰

Food & Water

8:15 a.m.	oatmeal, maple	6:00 p.m.	pill (2nd B-12)
8:30 a.m.	pills (1st B-12)	7:30 p.m.	talapia, broccoli,
10:45 a.m.	1st water done		lettuce, spinach
11:40 a.m.	2nd water done	8:00 p.m.	4th water done
12:45 p.m.	soup, crab	9:30 p.m.	chocolate chip cookie
3:30 p.m.	3rd water done	10:30 p.m.	chocolate bar
4:30 p.m.	chocolate bar		

Exercise

Run: 20 minutes w/dog.
Weights: bench press (wide), 3 sets; bench press (narrow), 3 sets; curls (bar), 3 sets.

Comments

I had an interesting discussion with my wife today. I reminded her that I have been thinking favorably about some meals I want to eat after I finish this diet program.

There are several foods I have been missing. Of course, that is with the condition that I consume only a moderate amount and that I offset the higher calories by a similar reduction at other meals in the same day.

Or that I will appropriately increase calorie-burning exercises in that day.

I have changed my mind, however. I don't mean that I am considering eating those meals recklessly. On the contrary. I am leaning toward avoiding them completely.

The reason is that I am worried. I have come a long way and worked very hard. I want nothing to spoil my success.

I do not want to regain even one pound. I just bought some new shirts. I like how they look and fit.

If I expand even a little, they will be worthless. I want them to last a long time.

I want to remain in top shape.

184

AFTER TWENTY WEEKS

IMPRESSIONS & PROGRESS

I almost quit! I had no thought of giving up on my weight-loss pursuit. I just considered finding another method.

A slight ascent in my weight had frustrated me. The point is moot, however.

I was turned back by weight loss. In the end, that is what it is all about.

So, it was just another hump in this emotional roller coaster.

In my self-prescribed therapy, I went and bought some new shirts. They are smaller than all my others, of course.

So, the pressure is on to ensure I never outgrow them. Having them fit well is a source of happiness.

Success thus far also has me rethinking my desire to enjoy a few meals from my pre-diet menu, once I complete the program.

I am hoping that desire fades to disappearance.

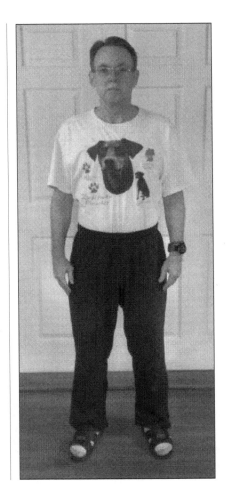

7

Success evidenced by taintless dreams

*W*e talk very little nowadays. As it should be, I suppose.

She has no meaningful words to offer. I have no questions. When we get together, we hurry to part ways.

The encounters have streamlined because my program is pretty much on "autopilot." My diet counselor watches as I step onto the scale. She records the latest number. Occasionally, she will measure me or have the computer perform a deeper analysis.

The minimum interaction means there are no glitches in the process. We are chugging along steadily toward the goal.

The only thing required now is patience. Sometimes I have a suitable amount.

Although I didn't see it as an interference or a speed bump, certain mental "occurrences" continue to puzzle me. My dreams have changed and I endeavor to understand them.

My dream scenarios for quite some time involved displaying some collection of events with me in the Navy. I get that.

I enjoyed many years in that outfit. The problem is that my dreams had constantly put me into an incorrect uniform. Certainly, back in the days of active duty, that would have caused me great trouble.

A U.S. Navy sailor simply does not wear the wrong shirt

or improper insignia. You do, of course, if you want to draw angry attention from persons in authority, which could lead to an unceremonious booting out of the service.

Obviously, none of those perils exist for this former sailor who merely has sleep-time visions of such situations.

But I am positive the dreams have a significant meaning. My wife has suggested they represent my frustration with my out-of-shape body.

This seems plausible—especially now that my Navy dreams no longer include me dressed in violation of regulations.

If you believe, as I do, that dreams are connected to something in the physical and conscious world of the dreamer, it is easy to conclude that some negative element of my life has been eliminated.

Frome there, it is but a small step, rather than a leap, to think that is a result of my body getting trimmed. I am quite happy with how I am shaping down.

And I do think of my new look frequently. Sigmund Freud, the famous psychiatrist, wrote that dreams are never complete fabrications. They all, he concluded, are connected to some recent item that was pondered in the conscious mind.

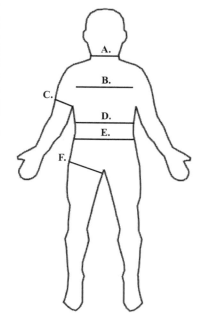

A. Neck: 15

B. Chest: 40.^{5}

C. Biceps: 12.^{5}

D. Waist (navel): 35

E. High Hip (belt line): 33

F. Thighs: 21

G. Weight: 156.^{0}

So, there is the connection to my weight loss. Even if I am wrong about this, two things are sure. My dreams have expelled the military uniform demons and my body is in significantly better condition.

My true mental foe is impatience.

I have given serious thought to quitting this program. While part of me is certain that sticking to it will allow me to achieve my weight-loss goal, another part questions the necessity of keeping on this course.

I know from past experience that I have the ability to lose weight by exercising vigorously and frequently. I must remember, however, that my own programs of the past have done nothing to make the weight loss permanent.

The fat, obviously, returned. Thus, I am hopeful this program will succeed where the others have failed.

So far, I can't argue that this is a completely different approach for me and it has been quite successful to this point.

Not too surprisingly, I will make no drastic changes just yet.

An alteration I have made, however, is my understanding of the end goal.

In recent weeks, I had what I call a "Rocky Balboa moment." That is when a flash of "brilliance" illuminates the situation and I realize a new direction may be desirable.

Part of my inspiration for diving into this particular program was a photograph of me when I was a skinny teenager. I thought, "Why can't I look like that again?" Well, that is a ridiculous idea—in totality. I never will look that young again.

I am not saying that was my actual intention. I just know that the best I can do is to be that thin again. That is definitely a challenging goal, but it is achievable.

To me, that realization is like Rocky understanding that his goal should not be to win but to get through all 12 rounds without getting beaten to unconsciousness.

He, a street-style slugger, after all, was going toe-to-toe with a world champion pugilist.

I would be battling father time, a greater impossibility than the one facing the "Italian Stallion."

So, my epipheny tells me to concentrate on hitting the right number of pounds and be set to appreciate that without having grander expectations.

Life will improve as a result. There is little doubt there. But elevating my hopes too high could be a recipe for catastrophe.

Day: #*141*   Weight: *156.⁰*

Food & Water

7:15 a.m.	oatmeal, blueberry	4:30 p.m.	pill (2nd B-12)
8:15 a.m.	pills (1st B-12)	5:30 p.m.	chocolate bar
9:15 a.m.	1st water done	8:30 p.m.	shrimp, scallops,
10:45 a.m.	soup, crab		broccoli, lettuce,
12:50 p.m.	2nd water done		spinach
2:15 p.m.	soup, chicken/rice	9:00 p.m.	4th water done
4:15 p.m.	3rd water done	10:00 p.m.	chocolate bar

Exercise

None today.

Comments

I had my weekly get-together with my program counselor. The short of it is that I have lost only one pound this past week. I lost little more than that the week before.

So, while I am not angry, I am questioning the value of continuing with the program now that I have lost a majority of the weight I need to lose.

Whether I really need to lose another 18 pounds is highly questionable.

Many of my friends look at me and say, "no way." They say my body can afford no more loss.

I am beginning to think they have a point. From a strictly monetary angle, I wonder whether it is worth what I pay for a week of food to shed a single pound.

In those terms, there is a good chance I will be shifting myself into my own program in the near future.

I am thinking about getting a second opinion from my doctor. I imagine he will say my current weight is fine and I should quit the diet, if that is my desire.

So, I will create a rough exit strategy.

Day: # *142*   Weight: *157.⁰*

Weight: $157.^0$

Food & Water

7:15 a.m.	eggs
8:00 a.m.	1st water done
8:20 a.m.	pills (1st B-12)
10:30 a.m.	soup, crab
10:45 a.m.	2nd water done
1:15 p.m.	soup, chicken/rice
5:30 p.m.	chocolate bar

7:30 p.m.	beef, broccoli, lettuce, spinach
8:00 p.m.	3rd water done
8:30 p.m.	pill (2nd B-12)
9:45 p.m.	chocolate chip cookie

Exercise

Run: 20 minutes w/dog.
Lower abs: bridges, 2 sets; leg raises, 2 sets.

Comments

Since I went to bed last night frustrated with my "slight" progress revealed at my weigh-in appointment, I had a less-than-nice dream about it and awoke at 4:30 a.m. feeling angry.

I was unable to get back to sleep. So, I got up, made and drank some coffee and checked my computer for the latest messages and other communications materials.

By 6 a.m., I was back on schedule and on my way to the work day.

In early afternoon, I ran into a coworker who completed this diet program last year.

He said he thought I already had achieved a great weight for my body.

He added that, if I felt I had arrived at a desirable weight, I should tell the program folks that I am happy with my body and want to shift to the "transition" stage.

I said I would seriously consider that approach. I will at least finish out the week and maybe get my doctor's opinion of my current status.

Day: #*143*   Weight: *156.⁶*

Food & Water

7:00 a.m.	eggs		5:00 p.m.	2nd water done
7:30 a.m.	pills (1st B-12)		7:30 p.m.	ground chicken,
9:30 a.m.	1st water done			broccoli, lettuce,
10:15 a.m.	soup, crab			spinach
1:15 p.m.	soup, chicken/rice		8:00 p.m.	3rd water done
4:30 p.m.	chocolate bar		9:30 p.m.	chocolate chip cookie
4:45 p.m.	pill (2nd B-12)			

Exercise

Swim: 20 laps (30 minutes).

Comments

Early in the day I was marveling at how my back seemed to be on the mend.

My level and frequency of discomfort has been way down. I even noted to myself how beneficial my swim seemed to have been.

When I hit the water, I had a sharp muscle pull on my left side that interfered with my stroke. Every time I stretched out my left arm I got a shooting pain.

As I pressed on and marked off a few laps, the pain almost vanished.

I figured the constant stretching took care of it.

As I sit at home and write this, I feel exhausted. I am thrilled with the level of work the swim required.

It didn't feel like much at the time I was doing it. But I know now that it whooped me.

I am ready for bed and it is only 9 p.m. Also, the comfort of my bed will rid me of this terrible pain in the middle of my back.

So, my nemesis has returned.

Drat!

Day: #*144*   Weight: *154.*⁸

Food & Water

7:15 a.m.	eggs
7:45 a.m.	pills (1st B-12)
9:45 a.m.	1st water done
10:30 a.m.	oatmeal, maple
1:30 p.m.	soup, crab
4:30 p.m.	chocolate bar
5:00 p.m.	2nd water done

7:30 p.m.	salmon, broccoli, lettuce, spinach
8:00 p.m.	3rd water done
8:15 p.m.	pill (2nd B-12)
10:20 p.m.	chocolate chip cookie

Exercise

Lower abs: bridges, 2 sets; leg raises, 2 sets.

Comments

Well, I don't normally use this space to refer to the day before. I must mention yesterday, though, as it has influenced my status today.

Specifically, I am referring to my swim. It had been months since I carved my way through the heated pool at a local community center.

Yesterday was my first day back at the activity. It felt pretty much the same, if you ignore the pulled muscle I had to overcome.

The level of energy I expended to complete my laps seemed similar to my past laps there.

Last night, however, I was spent. The swim did that.

I was much more tired than I have gotten on any recent run. The swim's beat-down impressed me enough to make me wonder how it could affect my calorie burn for the day.

When I hopped atop my bathroom scale, I got the answer. I was down more than a pound.

Maybe it was a fluke and I won't see that again. But I sure want to get back to the pool to find out.

193

Day: #*145*   Weight: *154.*²

Food & Water

8:30 a.m.	eggs
8:45 a.m.	pills (1st B-12)
9:30 a.m.	1st water done
11:45 a.m.	soup, crab
12:15 p.m.	2nd water done
2:30 p.m.	chocolate bar
5:30 p.m.	pill (2nd B-12)

5:45 p.m.	soup, chicken/rice
6:00 p.m.	3rd water done
9:00 p.m.	ground chicken, broccoli, lettuce, spinach
10:30 p.m.	chocolate chip cookie
10:45 p.m.	4th water done

Exercise

Swim: 20 laps (25 minutes).
Run: 20 minutes w/dog.

Weights: bench press (wide), 3 sets; bench press (narrow), 3 sets.

Comments

I am beat! I got a good swim in this morning. Then I took the kids on a four-mile trek at the beach boardwalk.

After that, the dog needed to run, so I obliged. After that, since I was good and warmed up, I hit the weights for about half of my upper body workout.

Certainly I had no need to work so hard today. But I am on a mission. I will do what it takes to reach my goal.

Right now, however, I am reexamining exactly what my goal should be. I doubt it is necessary or even feasible to arrive at the goal weight the program folks chose for me.

If I continue to drop some more pounds, I will press on, as long as it is fat burning away and not muscle.

Still, I am looking forward to moving off of the packaged diet meals and on to normal, healthful and low-calorie foods.

I am bothered because I looked at the literature on the "transition" plan. It calls for six more weeks of eating program foods while slowly adding some more veggies and some fruit. I am unsure whether that will be my plan.

Day: #*146*   Weight: *153.*⁶

Food & Water

8:45 a.m.	pills (1st B-12)		6:10 p.m.	2nd water done
9:00 a.m.	oatmeal, maple		7:30 p.m.	shrimp, scallops,
10:00 a.m.	1st water done			broccoli, zucchini,
11:45 a.m.	chocolate bar			lettuce, spinach
3:15 p.m.	sloppy joe		8:20 p.m.	3rd water done
5:55 p.m.	pill (2nd B-12)		9:30 p.m.	chocolate chip cookie
6:00 p.m.	mashed potatoes			

Exercise

Swim: 20 laps (26 minutes).

Comments

As I noted yesterday, it seems obvious that the swim is a top-notch calorie burner.

I was thinking of that for most of the day while the wife, kids and I walked around admiring all the entrants and guests at a local dog show.

After we got home in mid-afternoon, I grabbed my gear and headed for the pool. It was anything but picturesque today.

The sky was dark with clouds that rained onto me during several laps.

Although the pool is heated, it took me 12 lengths to get warm.

I was able to shave a few minutes from my usual time for 20 laps. That is a direct result of hitting the water more often.

Also, my mood is a little better today. I am not so negative on this diet program.

I am not, for the moment, demanding that I move beyond the packaged meal situation.

If I have a similar scale-response tomorrow as I had today, my attitude will remain enthusiastic.

If not, I suppose I will focus again on getting to the next step.

Day: #*147*   Weight: *152.*8

Food & Water

8:00 a.m.   eggs
8:15 a.m.   pills (1st B-12)
8:45 a.m.   1st water done
11:30 a.m.   soup, crab
1:15 p.m.   2nd water done
3:00 p.m.   soup, chicken/rice
4:30 p.m.   3rd water done

6:15 p.m.   pill (2nd B-12)
7:15 p.m.   ground chicken,
             broccoli, lettuce
8:15 p.m.   4th water done
9:30 p.m.   chocolate chip cookie
10:30 p.m.   chocolate bar

Exercise

None today.

Comments

Over the last few days, I have been focusing on severing my ties with this diet meal plan.

I really have been wanting to quit buying and eating the packaged meals and move on to more normal things to eat.

I only can guess why I was so headstrong about it. Oddly, today, however, I have pretty much reversed that thinking,

Today I see how it makes good sense to continue the pre-made meals while slowly introducing other foods into the lineup.

If I were to stop abruptly and make all my food from the grocery store shelves or restaurants, there is a good chance I would adopt many of my old eating habits.

That would jeopardize all that I have achieved in weight loss. I believe I am seeing the wisdom of the plan because I have found some peace of mind through the luxurious exercise called swimming.

It really is mentally therapeutic. I had forgotten what a great feeling I have while swimming and for hours afterward.

It truly is remarkable.

21

Total pounds lost so far:

54.²

AFTER TWENTY-ONE WEEKS

IMPRESSIONS & PROGRESS

Do I really need to lose 18 pounds more? That is what I wondered just days ago.

My friends seem to think I am through with this diet thing. They told me so.

They note with tongue firmly in cheek, "You're disappearing. Have a sandwich or something."

It is difficult to make such an assessment myself. I have relied on family and serious coworkers. I also feel my body is a big controller in the matter.

I am in no way starving. So, whether another 18 pounds must go is debatable, but I see no reason to put on the brakes just yet.

I will verify with my doctor, of course.

Since I am pressing on, my workout has expanded to include a dunk in the pool. Swimming again is a great joy.

It is excellent exercise that also is mentally therapeutic. Life is good.

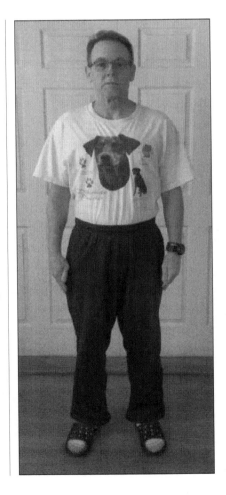

197

Day: #*148*   Weight: *153.*²

Food & Water

7:15 a.m.	oatmeal, blueberry
7:30 a.m.	pills (1st B-12)
8:45 a.m.	1st water done
11:00 a.m.	soup, crab
1:15 p.m.	2nd water done
2:45 p.m.	soup, chicken/rice
4:15 p.m.	3rd water done
8:30 p.m.	ground chicken, broccoli, lettuce, spinach
9:00 p.m.	4th water done
9:30 p.m.	chocolate chip cookie
10:00 p.m.	chocolate bar

Exercise

None today.

Comments

I had a bit of a shock today. Chasing an itch, I reached for my back to scratch it. My fingers found bone.

It was my shoulder blade. What a surprise! I don't think I have felt that in many years.

I suppose if I let my fingers walk around my body, they will find other, similar results.

At first glance, it would seem this is good evidence of success in a fat-burning program. And it is.

My second thought, however, was about limits. Have I exceeded one? Am I getting too skinny?

How will I know when to stop? My history with body weight shows I am a poor judge in this area.

I also don't want to develop a mental problem where, no matter how thin I get, I still think I am fat.

That would be disastrous.

So, I asked my wife. She says I am fine, that I shouldn't worry. Okay, I am going to confirm that with my doctor.

I have an appointment to discuss some things with him and I will get that needed professional opinion.

Day: #*149*   Weight: *153.*[6]

Food & Water

7:30 a.m.	eggs
8:20 a.m.	pills (1st B-12)
9:45 a.m.	1st water done
10:30 a.m.	soup, crab
1:00 p.m.	2nd water done
1:30 p.m.	soup, chicken/rice
4:00 p.m.	pill (2nd B-12)

4:30 p.m.	oatmeal, blueberry
7:30 p.m.	salmon, lettuce, broccoli, zucchini
8:15 p.m.	3rd water done
10:00 p.m.	chocolate bar

Exercise

Swim: 20 laps (26 minutes). Weights: bench press, 3 sets; curls (bar), 3 sets; curls (bells), 3 sets.

Comments

I had a conversation today with a coworker about dieting, eating in general and resulting bodies.

It was the same coworker I spoke to weeks ago about this diet program. He was interested because he wanted to lose about 15 or 20 pounds, I think.

He has made no call yet for a free consultation. I was talking about how I am going to be very hesitant about eating "normal" food again because I don't want to reverse any of the success I have achieved on this diet.

I said I still have a bit of body fat to expel but don't want to obsess about it. He told me about a couple of guys he worked with years ago.

They were body builders and never would go with a work group to restaurants because the menus had nothing they could eat.

My coworker said he never wants to be like that. I agreed that's an extreme. But reality for people who don't want to bloat with body fat is not too far from that position.

Restaurant food has that effect and must be handled appropriately to limit its damage.

Day: #*150*   Weight: *152.*⁶

Food & Water

7:15 a.m.	oatmeal, blueberry
7:30 a.m.	pills (1st B-12)
7:45 a.m.	1st water done
10:30 a.m.	soup, crab
1:45 p.m.	soup, chicken/rice
4:15 p.m.	2nd water done
4:45 p.m.	chocolate bar

7:30 p.m.	beef, broccoli, lettuce, spinach
8:40 p.m.	3rd water done
9:20 p.m.	pill (2nd B-12)
9:35 p.m.	chocolate chip cookie

Exercise

Swim: 20 laps (30 minutes).

Comments

Today was a big day. I saw my doctor. I felt it was time to have blood tests done again to see if my bad cholesterol levels were down to normal now that I have shed more than 50 pounds.

It has been so long since I did that test I forgot I must fast for at least 10 hours prior to my blood getting extracted.

So, I must return in the morning for that. But the big news of the day was my doctor's confirmation that I am a good weight for my height right now.

He said that, if I continued and lost a few more pounds, I would not be too skinny. He also said that today I am not overweight.

When I told him the goal weight the program had set for me, he said, "One-hundred-forty-two! Really?" Then, he added, "Hey, you know they have a financial incentive for setting a very low goal weight?"

I acknowledged and noted I already had surpassed my own initial goal weight.

In the end, I would like to drop five more pounds to make it an even 60 lost.

I can do that while I transition off of their packaged foods.

Day: #*151*   Weight: *152.⁰*

Food & Water

8:30 a.m.	eggs		7:30 p.m.	talapia, lettuce, broccoli, spinach
9:15 a.m.	pills (1st B-12)		8:00 p.m.	3rd water done
9:30 a.m.	1st water done		8:45 p.m.	pill (2nd B-12)
10:45 a.m.	soup, crab		10:00 p.m.	chocolate chip cookie
1:45 p.m.	soup, chicken/rice			
2:00 p.m.	2nd water done			
4:30 p.m.	oatmeal, maple			

Exercise

Swim: 20 laps (25 minutes).

Comments

Today was filled with enthusiasm. I probably had more than my share, however.

I was able to get to the pool at lunch break from work. The weather was good, the water warm.

I normally mix my strokes, one lap crawl, the next breast stroke, etc.

I alternate because I am not in top condition since I took so much time off from this specific exercise.

But today I felt great and figured I should maximize the number of freestyle-stroke laps.

My leaking new goggles helped. They made me stop briefly at the end of each lap to empty and realign them.

It turned out that all my laps but one were of the crawl variety. When I touched the coping at the tail of my 20th lap, I felt no different, physically.

Mentally, I was beaming.

My body reminded me later that I am no longer young and need to make such stress increases at a more gradual pace. Another lesson was learned.

I should say it was "reintroduced" to me.

Day: #*152*   Weight: *151.*⁴

Food & Water

7:30 a.m.	eggs		5:30 p.m.	sloppy joe
8:10 a.m.	pills (1st B-12)		6:30 p.m.	3rd water done
9:30 a.m.	1st water done		9:00 p.m.	ground chicken,
10:45 a.m.	soup, crab			broccoli, lettuce,
11:15 a.m.	2nd water done			spinach
2:00 p.m.	soup, chicken/rice		10:00 p.m.	4th water done
5:00 p.m.	pill (2nd B-12)		11:30 p.m.	chocolate bar

Exercise

Swim: 20 laps (30 minutes).

Comments

I believe I have made a decision. It concerns my goal weight.

I know I have noted numerous times that I am eager to conclude the program meal plan and get on with life. Of course, a plan for exactly when and how I should do that has not presented itself.

But, I think I have it now. Since I am adjusting my goal weight to 147, I am now about four-and-a-half pounds away.

I am continuing to lose weight and expect to be even closer to goal in the morning. So, if I begin the transition in three days, when I have my next appointment with my counselor, I should be extremely close. Then I will have the first week of transitioning without a significant change to my meal schedule.

I feel strongly that the slight alteration in my diet then will have no adverse effect on my continued weight loss and I will achieve my goal weight before moving fully away from the packaged meals and adopting a full-calorie load for my normal existence.

The goal weight set for me by the program was unnecessarily low and will not be missed... well, figuratively, that is.

Day: #*153*   Weight: *152.⁰*

Food & Water

7:30 a.m.	oatmeal, maple
7:45 a.m.	pills (1st B-12)
8:30 a.m.	1st water done
10:45 a.m.	soup, crab
11:00 a.m.	2nd water done
3:15 p.m.	soup, chicken/rice
3:30 p.m.	pill (2nd B-12)

5:00 p.m.	3rd water done
7:30 p.m.	salmon, lettuce, broccoli
9:00 p.m.	4th water done
9:30 p.m.	cappuccino (decaf)
11:00 p.m.	chocolate bar

Exercise

Weights: squats, 3 sets; calf raises, 3 sets.

Swim: 20 laps (28 minutes).

Comments

Today tested my mettle.

It was cold and rainy. Although it is the weekend and I could have aimed myself toward the pool at any time, there would be no break in the crappy weather.

So, it was in the lunch hour as usual that I packed my gear and drove off to the community center.

I moved briskly across the deck (slowly enough to avoid a lifeguard's whistle) on my way to the locker room.

I didn't mind the rain so much. I was there to get wet. But I have a low tolerance for the cold.

So, I was thrilled to feel the warm water envelop me as I dropped myself into the blue.

What a cozy and satisfying feeling that was. I really didn't want to leave the water.

I had company. Two other people were carving lanes nearby. Maybe they were on a mission as well.

When I had endured enough, I bounced to the locker room, changed, moseyed contentedly along the route back to my car.

I gave a thankful wave to the lifeguards for keeping an eye on the diehards at play.

Day: #*154*   Weight: *150.⁶*

Food & Water

7:15 a.m.	eggs
8:05 a.m.	pills (1st B-12)
8:20 a.m.	1st water done
11:20 a.m.	chocolate bar
2:45 p.m.	soup, crab
3:30 p.m.	2nd water done
4:00 p.m.	pill (2nd B-12)

5:45 p.m.	chocolate bar
7:15 p.m.	pork, broccoli, lettuce
8:00 p.m.	3rd water done
9:45 p.m.	chocolate bar

Exercise

Swim: 20 laps (25 minutes).

Comments

My swim today was very interesting. The sun peeked through the clouds as I made my way over to a metal bleacher to set my gear on while I was in the water.

As I passed the lifeguard, he said my timing was great. They had just let people back into the pool after evacuating it because of thunder.

It had just rained. Benches and chairs were soaked. I could see some black clouds tangled with some puffy white ones.

The air was chilly, but the water was comfortable.

All of that may have been interesting , but it was not why I described my outing that way. The reason for that came upon my exit from the blue.

I was walking back to my bag and towel when I passed a chain of mirrored windows. My swim shirt was clinging to my soaked form and I saw a small but distinct roll of fat at my belt line.

"Oh, my..." I thought. "Look at that!"

I guess I need to burn some more calories. Should I postpone my transition off of the program? Or is that me obsessing?

AFTER TWENTY-TWO WEEKS

IMPRESSIONS & PROGRESS

I can see my ribs! That vision has escaped me for decades.

That bone collection seems to be holding up fairly well.

I also found my shoulder bones have become visible. Am I shriveling up?

I finally got my doctor to weigh in on my physique. Weigh in? Did I need to use that verb?

Anyway, he said I am fine. Losing some more fat would not make me too thin. Also, staying as I am is okay as well. So, that issue is settled.

I will continue, at least for a bit. But I have identified the date I will begin my transition to non-packaged meals.

At that point, I will accept whatever the scale reads for me. It still will be possible to lose a few more pounds during the weeks of the changeover, however.

So, I may not have reached my final weight when I jump to a new menu.

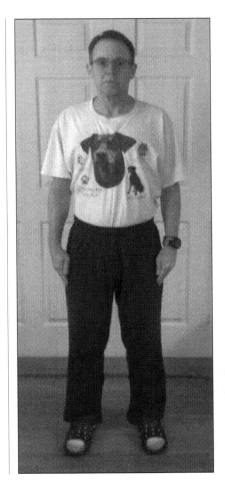

Day: #*155*   Weight: *150.*^6^

Food & Water

7:00 a.m.	eggs
7:45 a.m.	pills (1st B-12)
8:55 a.m.	1st water done
10:45 a.m.	soup, crab
2:15 p.m.	soup, chicken/rice
2:30 p.m.	2nd water done
4:45 p.m.	pill (2nd B-12)

5:15 p.m.	chocolate bar
7:45 p.m.	ground chicken, broccoli, lettuce, spinach
8:30 p.m.	3rd water done
10:15 p.m.	chocolate bar

Exercise

Swim: 25 laps (29 minutes).

Comments

Well, today was another interesting day in my dilemma about when to pull the plug on my diet program.

I went to my appointment and got weighed. I got no order to remove my socks for the machine to analyze me.

That was to be my indicator that they didn't want to bother. I suspected because they didn't want me to see I was burning muscle, which would cause me to quit now.

As I left the scale and headed to my shoes, my counselor asked if I wanted to get the analysis today or wait until next week.

I peeled off my socks and climbed aboard. When we received the results, I learned that I had lost 11.4 pounds of body fat, but only 9 pounds of weight. That means I built muscle and burned fat.

All is very well.

So, I decided to stick with it another week or so to drop the last three pounds to reach MY goal.

I was feeling so good that I swam a greater distance at a faster pace than usual.

I am beat but happy as I write this in my log.

Day: #156   Weight: 150.^{6}

Food & Water

8:00 a.m.	oatmeal, maple		6:30 p.m.	pill (2nd B-12)
8:15 a.m.	pills (1st B-12)		7:30 p.m.	talapia, lettuce, broccoli, spinach
10:20 a.m.	1st water done		8:15 p.m.	3rd water done
11:00 a.m.	soup, crab		9:00 p.m.	4th water done
2:00 p.m.	chocolate bar		10:00 p.m.	chocolate bar
4:10 p.m.	2nd water done			
5:15 p.m.	mashed potatoes			

Exercise

None today.

Comments

Well, today was quite a letdown. I suppose I could say I should have expected as much, since the day began with a frozen scale.

By that I mean its reading was stuck on the number it displayed yesterday. It was no mechanical or electrical malfunction.

It was telling me my weight had remained unchanged.

But no, that was not the culprit. Work activities and a board meeting consumed my time and prohibited me from getting to the pool for a swim.

Of course, work comes first. It makes so many things possible and I am free to realign my events outside of work so I can hit the water at an alternate time.

But this day refused to allow that. And I got involved in things at home, so a replacement exercise remained elusive as well.

So, I am feeling a bit gloomy. Part of that is from guilt. Another portion is a result of not having enjoyed that warm water and the luxurious muscle strain that comes from 20 laps in the sunshine.

I am looking forward to tomorrow.

Day: #*157* Weight: *150.²*

Food & Water

7:00 a.m.   oatmeal, maple
7:45 a.m.   pills (1st B-12)
10:00 a.m. 1st water done
10:30 a.m. soup, crab
1:45 p.m.   soup, chicken/rice
2:00 p.m.   2nd water done
5:00 p.m.   chocolate bar

6:30 p.m.   pill (2nd B-12)
7:30 p.m.   pork, broccoli, lettuce, spinach
8:00 p.m.   3rd water done
9:45 p.m.   chocolate bar

Exercise

Swim: 20 laps (23.5 minutes).
Run: 15 minutes (w/dog).

Weights: bench press, 3 sets; curls (bar), 3 sets.

Comments

I was in beast mode today.

Not only did I swim all laps with a crawl stroke, I pushed it and cut my time.

It felt good and the water was awesome as usual. Then, later at home, I pulled on my sneakers, stretched out, leashed the mutt and dashed through the neighborhood on a run.

The dash was less than stellar. As I was pounding the pavement, I thought again of racing and how I am so far from fit for competition.

My swimming has improved quickly. The run is still a difficult drag, however. Maybe, if I push it like I have my swim, I will feel some improvement being made.

It is not that I really expect to enjoy jogging, but I should feel more energetic, at least.

After that mediocre event, I lifted weights. That always gives me a good boost because I can feel the work focused on specific muscles and it seems the benefit is more apparent as I raise the weight.

All in all, though, it was a very good day.

Day: #*158*   Weight: *149.*^8

Food & Water

7:00 a.m.	eggs		4:15 p.m.	oatmeal, maple
8:30 a.m.	pills (1st B-12)		4:20 p.m.	pill (2nd B-12)
9:15 a.m.	1st water done		7:30 p.m.	ground chicken,
10:15 a.m.	soup, crab			lettuce, broccoli,
11:15 a.m.	2nd water done			spinach, zucchini
1:15 p.m.	soup, chicken/rice		8:25 p.m.	4th water done
1:35 p.m.	3rd water done		9:30 p.m.	chocolate bar

Exercise

Swim: 20 laps (26 minutes).

Comments

Yeehaw! My weight dipped below 150 this morning. It only slightly crossed the line, but that is a major step for me.

I literally have not been this light since I was a teenager. Avoiding embarrassing precision, I will round that out to more than 30 years ago.

So, yes, I am excited. I am thrilled to be so close to my goal. And, thus, the temptations that present themselves are even easier to ignore.

I had another such test today in my workplace lounge. A coworker was celebrating her birthday. So she baked and brought to share some "monkey bread" and a raspberry cream cheese coffee cake.

No one seemed to know how the bread got its name as they picked it apart with their fingers and ran to other parts of the room to enjoy it privately.

The basic name of the cake was fitting but couldn't begin to communicate the awesomeness of the aroma that drifted above the luxurious, textured surface.

Everyone who tasted it said it was "dreamy." I am unable to argue that, but my perspective was limited to smell. And that was enough.

Day: #*159*   Weight: *148.*⁴

Food & Water

8:15 a.m.	oatmeal, maple
8:40 a.m.	pills (1st B-12)
11:45 a.m.	soup, crab
12:05 p.m.	1st water done
5:05 p.m.	chocolate bar
5:15 p.m.	2nd water done
5:45 p.m.	pill (2nd B-12)

8:30 p.m.	ground chicken, broccoli, lettuce, spinach
9:20 p.m.	3rd water done
10:15 p.m.	chocolate chip cookie
10:45 p.m.	chocolate bar

Exercise

Swim: 20 laps (26 minutes).

Comments

The highlight of my day was my swim. That should be no surprise to anyone. There was a guy there who seemed set on disturbing my tranquility, however.

There were numerous lanes open, but he plopped into one right next to me. That normally would have no meaning. This guy, though, flailed.

I called him "The Splasher" in my thoughts. His wake slapped me around quite a bit. It was no big deal, really, and I bid him a silent and friendly farewell when the lane on my other side opened and I slid into it.

The next obstacle came in the locker room. While changing back to my street clothes, I saw myself in a mirror.

I have trimmed down plenty, but I have two distinct bags of fat hanging on my chest. They dangle from the top front of my rib cage.

"How can I get rid of those?" I thought. I am burning fat but there it remains. My mind wandered to... "liposuction!"

You have got to be kidding, I thought. Has it come to this?

Well, I don't believe I was serious. That is extreme... isn't it?

Day: # *160*   Weight: *148.*²

Food & Water

9:00 a.m.	oatmeal, maple
9:45 a.m.	pills (1st B-12)
11:30 a.m.	1st water done
1:00 p.m.	soup, crab
1:30 p.m.	2nd water done
3:45 p.m.	chocolate bar
6:30 p.m.	pill (2nd B-12)

7:30 p.m.	salmon, lettuce, broccoli, spinach,
8:00 p.m.	3rd water done
9:00 p.m.	chocolate chip cookie
10:00 p.m.	chocolate bar

Exercise

Run: 20 minutes (w/dog).

Comments

I consciously reminded myself today that I am getting pretty disinterested in writing down everything I eat and drink.

I know it has been an essential part of the program. I am just very close to the end and it is becoming a boring chore.

Speaking of nearing completion, I had a wild idea today to verify my height. There was little question about that until my doctor seemed to confirm my suspicions.

For years, I have been 5'7". my diet counselor measured me at 5'6". No alarm sounded. I expected it. I am aging, after all.

So, today, I marked a wall level with the top of my noggin, stretched the tape and found I had experienced no significant shrinkage.

You could look at it as a quarter-inch lower, but not a full inch. Why is this meaningful? Well, the ideal weight for me at the lower height is six pounds away.

At the taller level, I am within two pounds of the ideal weight. With a lower goal weight, the program gets me to buy more food from them.

Could that have influenced their eyesight when measuring?

Day: #*161*   Weight: *148.²*

Food & Water

8:00 a.m.	oatmeal, maple
9:00 a.m.	pills (1st B-12)
11:00 a.m.	1st water done
1:15 p.m.	soup, crab
3:00 p.m.	2nd water done
4:15 p.m.	chocolate bar
4:45 p.m.	3rd water done

7:00 p.m.	pill (2nd B-12)
7:45 p.m.	talapia, spinach
	broccoli, lettuce,
8:15 p.m.	4th water done
9:45 p.m.	chocolate chip cookie
10:20 p.m.	chocolate bar

Exercise

Swim: 20 laps (25 minutes).

Comments

I got a late start on meals today. Actually, it is more accurate to say my second meal was delayed a couple of hours.

That pushed things back and found me quite hungry around the time my "normal" dinner was in the works.

It was not an earth-shattering experience, but it reminded me of the importance of spreading out the meals as equally as possible throughout the day.

The body and mind will be thankful. I also had an idea to help myself stay on the right path for thinness and good health.

I chose to write this book for the same reason: to keep me moving forward with an additional goal to enjoy at the end of the road.

So, another writing project is needed to help continue the success. I will create and maintain a blog on the internet. I will research, write and share articles on exercise and nutrition.

Readers can comment and share their opinions and knowledge so none of us has to go it alone.

We can keep an eye on each other and provide encouragement. It appears to be a plan.

23

Total pounds lost so far: 58.⁸

AFTER TWENTY-THREE WEEKS

IMPRESSIONS & PROGRESS

I reached a milestone this week. my weight sunk below 150 pounds. I have been heavier than that (significantly) since I was a teenager.

That was decades ago. I never would have believed it possible to enjoy this build again.

But I also am not done!

Partly because I am happy and partly to help me keep nutrition and fitness perpetually in my conscious mind, I have decided to create and maintain a blog on the subjects.

The web address will be **FlablesslyFit.com**. As I research for food and exercise information, publishing my findings there will allow me to share important facts with others who are trying to get, or stay, in shape.

The site's corresponding social media addresses will be **Facebook.com/FlablesslyFit** and **@FlablesslyFit** (Twitter). Those will permit people to share their info and success stories, too.

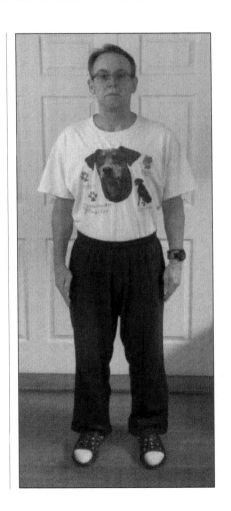

Day: #*162*   Weight: *148.²*

Food & Water

7:30 a.m.	oatmeal, maple		4:35 p.m.	sloppy joe
8:35 a.m.	pills (1st B-12)		5:00 p.m.	3rd water done
9:15 a.m.	1st water done		8:00 p.m.	ground chicken,
10:45 a.m.	soup, crab			broccoli, lettuce,
1:45 p.m.	soup, chicken/rice			spinach
2:35 p.m.	2nd water done		8:30 p.m.	4th water done
4:15 p.m.	pill (2nd B-12)		10:00 p.m.	chocolate bar

Exercise

Swim: 20 laps (25 minutes).

Comments

The breakup was a tad awkward. "It's not you," I said. "It's me."

I let them know today that I had only two or so more pounds to drop to reach *MY* goal.

I said I would not be shooting for the goal they had set for me, which is about nine pounds away, according to their scale.

They informed me of a benefit I would be eligible for, if I were to continue and reach their goal weight: a 10 percent discount on the purchase of their food forever.

I declined.

I think I can get that food anytime on the internet cheaper than theirs even with their "sale" price.

More importantly, my plan is to stay in shape and never need them or their packaged offerings again.

For good measure (terrible pun), I added that their goal weight for me should have been higher since I am actually 5-foot-7 rather than 5-foot-6, as they recorded my height.

They checked again with the same result.

Anyhow, we will be seeing less of each other soon.

Day: #*163*   Weight: *149.⁰*

Food & Water

7:30 a.m.	eggs	4:45 p.m.	pill (2nd B-12)
8:00 a.m.	pills (1st B-12)	7:30 p.m.	salmon, lettuce,
9:30 a.m.	1st water done		broccoli, spinach,
10:45 a.m.	soup, crab	7:45 p.m.	3rd water done
1:30 p.m.	soup, chicken/rice	11:00 p.m.	chocolate bar
1:45 p.m.	2nd water done		
4:30 p.m.	chocolate bar		

Exercise

None today.

Comments

Okay, I must admit: I felt some fear today.

I weighed in this morning almost a pound up from yesterday.

I know. That means nothing. The ups and downs have been with me since the diet began.

But now I am ready to pull the plug when I am but a couple of pounds from my target.

I am worried I will fail to shed the last pound and cross the finish line.

I also am feeling like an extra few pounds' loss would be a good buffer in case my weight bounces up for some reason after I reach my goal.

So, although I am very eager to move on, I am going to be patient.

I will make no drastic moves until I am sure I have hit my goal weight and feel comfortable pitching in the towel.

Of course, I will begin a new plan for eating properly and exercising right so I maintain the new body.

I just have to make the timing absolutely on the mark.

215

Day: #*164*   Weight: *149.⁰*

Food & Water

7:15 a.m.	eggs
8:30 a.m.	pills (1st B-12)
9:05 a.m.	1st water done
10:45 a.m.	soup, crab
1:00 p.m.	2nd water done
1:45 p.m.	soup, chicken/rice
3:50 p.m.	pill (2nd B-12)
4:05 p.m.	3rd water done
4:40 p.m.	chocolate bar
7:15 p.m.	shrimp, spinach broccoli, lettuce
8:30 p.m.	4th water done
10:00 p.m.	chocolate bar

Exercise

Swim: 20 laps (23.5 minutes).

Comments

I am in conflict. I saw my reflection again at the pool. My swim trunks' drawstring created a small roll of flesh at the belt line.

It made me look harder at the rest of my midsection. I realized I could lose a few more pounds there.

My head still is residing in reality, however, as I also realize losing more is unnecessary. But that is why I am torn.

As soon as I break from the diet, I will not jump back on to try to drop a couple more. So, I am warming up to the idea of continuing a bit longer.

This decision bothers no one.

I must be careful, though, as I do not want to get fixated on getting even skinnier.

That could develop into an unhealthy state of mind. To help myself stay committed to my newfound slenderness, I am investing in new clothes.

It would hurt me greatly to outgrow them. They will constantly remind me to keep eating right and exercising.

And maybe I should quit looking at my image in full-length mirrors.

Day: # *165*　　　　Weight: *148.*⁴

Food & Water

7:15 a.m.	eggs
8:00 a.m.	pills (1st B-12)
9:30 a.m.	1st water done
10:30 a.m.	soup, crab
1:45 p.m.	soup, chicken/rice
2:00 p.m.	2nd water done
4:30 p.m.	chocolate bar
4:45 p.m.	pill (2nd B-12)
7:15 p.m.	chicken, lettuce, broccoli, spinach,
8:00 p.m.	3rd water done
10:15 p.m.	chocolate chip cookie

Exercise

Swim: 20 laps (23.5 minutes).

Comments

Donuts in the lounge! This time I wanted one. I tasted it... a luscious, round, chocolate-covered beauty.

My mouth watered as I smelled the aroma. The taste, fortunately, was only in my mind.

The notable thing to me was that I actually wanted to eat it. I gave it no deliberation. I gave no consideration to having just a bite.

I walked away quickly. Still, after 164 days of great success and mental fortitude, my knees wobbled in the face of the enemy.

I need to circle the chuck wagons and decide how to get back to having no interest in those fat pills.

I worry that, one day, after the hard core diet is done, I might think one bite won't hurt. Then, one donut won't hurt.

That begins the spiral. It also begs the thought, "Why can't a person of good health and body have a donut?" The answer: "You should be able to enjoy one now and then without issue."

So, how to do that without suffering a mental battle at each encounter? And how to ensure "occasionally" doesn't become "routine."

I will ponder this dilemma during my swim.

Day: #*166*   Weight: *147.*⁶

Food & Water

7:30 a.m.	eggs		5:55 p.m.	3rd water done
8:15 a.m.	pills (1st B-12)		9:15 p.m.	ground chicken,
8:30 a.m.	1st water done			spinach, zucchini
11:40 a.m.	soup, crab			broccoli, lettuce
12:55 p.m.	2nd water done		9:40 p.m.	4th water done
5:20 p.m.	soup, chicken/rice		10:30 p.m.	chocolate bar
5:50 p.m.	pill (2nd B-12)			

Exercise

Swim: 20 laps (25 minutes).

Comments

Big news today! My scale was kind this morning. I had a few days of depressing progress. Make that "no" progress.

But now I am about half-a-pound from my goal weight. It is almost time to celebrate.

For the rest of today, however, I need to get on with my routine.

I rechecked my height. My counselor was right. I am 5-foot-6. I guess that has no effect on my goal weight.

It does confirm their measurement and validates the goal weight they selected for me. That was about four pounds different from what it would have been, if I were still 5-foot-7.

I am glad to set the record straight and clear their measuring device from suspicion.

Big news today! ...It is almost time to celebrate.

Day: #*167*   Weight: *146.*^6

Food & Water

8:30 a.m.	eggs
8:45 a.m.	pills (1st B-12)
9:10 a.m.	1st water done
11:30 a.m.	soup, crab
11:55 a.m.	2nd water done
2:45 p.m.	soup, chicken/rice
7:00 p.m.	3rd water done

7:25 p.m.	pill (2nd B-12)
8:00 p.m.	beef, lettuce, broccoli, spinach,
9:15 p.m.	4th water done
10:00 p.m.	chocolate bar
10:05 p.m.	chocolate bar

Exercise

Swim: 20 laps (23.5 minutes).

Comments

Goooooaaaaaaalllll...! I did it. I surpassed 60 pounds. That is a lot of weight gone... nearly one-third of my body.

It is a day to celebrate. Not with cake, though. I probably will just swim and enjoy the knowledge that it has been a long road to get here.

And I know the journey is anything but over. I will make some adjustments, but the focus must remain so I can maintain good health and eating habits.

Well, I must get on with this big day. The rest of the day included a shopping trip to several stores. It was no shopping "spree" mind you. It persisted because I had trouble finding the right dress shirt in my size. I also needed slim-fit undershirts so they won't bunch up beneath the see-through outer garment.

In this search, I discovered that boys' size XL is much the same as men's small, revealing a far less expensive option for some future purchases.

We concluded our trip when we found a couple of no-iron fitted dress shirts in my size.

My lovely wife surprised me by adding an awesome and bright tie as a gift from her to mark my achievement.

8

Goal weight achieved! What now?

*I*n the "transition" period, I was "itching" to get to regular food. As with the entire program, however, patience was imperative.

Also, as with the full program, I didn't know that until I had completed it.

Forcing it to be stretched over four to six weeks kept me from stumbling because I was "running" too fast.

Working non-packaged meals into the daily lineup one-at-a-time was a benefit. It helped me to remain accurate in my calorie count and intake.

Of course, I kept telling myself, "I don't need to coast along on training wheels. I can handle the downhill zip-speed on my own."

The truth of that I will never know because I stuck to the program and followed the rules. I am satisfied with the outcome and, therefore, recommend adhering to the plan.

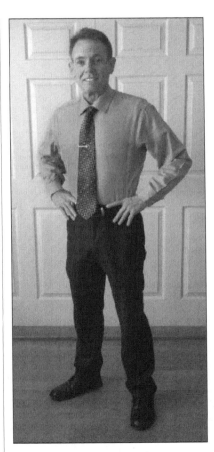

* I continued to lose weight during my transition to all regular food.

221

Reaching the point of transitioning meant the official diet program had ended. The weight loss and responsibilities, however, continued.

I lost several more pounds, reaching 139. That's 68 pounds down as a result of this diet program.

Overall, I am 80 pounds lower than my worst point. While the scale bounces up and down a pound or two above and below (will that ever stop?), I have maintained that level for months since moving on to a "normal" eating routine.

I guess this is a pivotal point. With the freedom to eat without a specific menu dictated by others, it could be easy to go astray.

This would be the spot where a dieter could fail and return to bad habits. I will admit, however, that I am so happy with my new (renewed) body—and so scared of overeating—that I doubt I will have any trouble staying fit.

I am pretty meticulous about counting the calories I consume, never exceeding the proper amount required to keep my weight under control.

Probably the single most important factor in predicting continued success, I think, is the level of education about food I have obtained from this diet program.

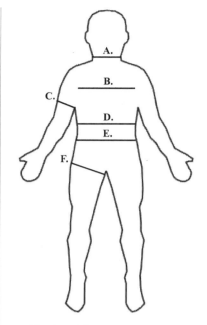

A. Neck: 14.^{5}

B. Chest: 38.^{5}

C. Biceps: 12.^{5}

D. Waist (navel): 31.^{5}

E. High Hip (belt line): 31

F. Thighs: 20.^{5}

G. Weight: 140.^{5}

My nutritionist and the printed materials she provided have given me the knowledge to be discriminating in my food choices.

That will ensure I am not mistakenly chomping down something that is horrendously bad for weight and health maintenance.

I also have learned, through a keen eye for detail and a renewed attentiveness, to ask the right questions. I have discovered how perilous the average restaurant is for anyone trying to avoid becoming obese.

When you insist on seeing the calorie content of entrees offered on the menu, you realize just how horrific those meals are.

In one of my old-favorite eateries, for example, I found an alarming fact. The cobb salad I previously gobbled while trying to be "good" (it's a salad, right?), contains about 1,200 calories.

That plate alone amounted to two-thirds of the recommended calories for my entire day. Add that to the reckless eating I did over the remaining hours before bedtime and it is easy to see how I packed on the pounds.

That doesn't mean that all restaurants, or all their meals, are bad.

With my new knowledge, I easily have navigated myself to new habits. I have zeroed-in on great-tasting meals that have a tolerable number of calories.

In fact, the casual calorie-hunter can find several family restaurants with low-calorie sections on their menus, offering quite palatable and filling meals.

At about 600 or fewer calories, those meals fit well into my new daily schedule, and they're not so high that they can't be countered easily with other choices that round out the day's consumption.

So, I have not had to steer entirely clear of commercial meal houses. Visits to them just need to be planned and dealt with appropriately.

Good thing, too. I doubt a person could survive in our society while trying to completely refrain from patronizing restaurants. They are a big part of our culture.

A little effort on the part of the dieter or health-conscious person makes them quite doable.

One of the interesting things about having lost so much weight is that it has made me much more conscious about weight control in general. Everywhere I look, I see obesity. It appears to be an epidemic. I hope this doesn't impress the reader in a way that it does when a person quits smoking and then attacks everyone else who still suffers from the habit.

On the contrary, I still understand obesity, how it is achieved and, most importantly, how to abolish it.

I also continue to empathize

with those who have been unable to kick it and continue to suffer its effects.

Oddly, I have heard from people who have struggled and failed on diets—yet they found plenty of energy to attack and criticize the program that worked so well for me and so many others.

I am unable to comprehend. I suppose it is a psychological defense maneuver. Or maybe a personality blemish is to blame.

Regardless, I refuse to waste any brain time trying to figure it out. The answer, even if attainable, is unlikely to benefit anyone.

My casual attitude is no accident. Another byproduct of being in such great shape is a calm that had escaped me in recent years.

While I was packing on the extra pounds and my body outline was seriously disproportioned, I lived with an enormous irritability.

I got angry for nothing. I could explode over almost anything. And, at the time, I had no idea I was so sensitive to minor stimuli.

My renewed sense of calm was one of the first things my wife noticed—after the normal figure I sported, of course.

She only could shake her head previously in reaction to my outbursts.

I would like to say I have gained an ability to face problems and tackle them with little effort. But that would be an overstatement.

Reality is that all those things I saw as problems were anything but. They were nothing to cause concern. Yet, I reacted in a way that gave them great power over me.

They rattled me.

It was an unearned status on their part. They deserved little, if any, attention. I promoted them to an undeserved rank in my life.

I hope never to do that again. I think I can control that by maintaining proper weight and routinely exercising to support good circulation. Blood flow assists mood, I am convinced.

My experience proves it to me, even if medical science may be unable to commit to it.

Another valuable benefit of success in this diet program is that many mysterious body pains have disappeared.

One known ailment has departed and I expect I never will suffer from it again.

For quite a long time, acid reflux hammered me. I took a pill every day to combat it.

Now that I am thin, the digestive juice remains where

it belongs. Since I drastically changed my body, acid no longer creeps up to scorch my throat.

With my new good moods, I contemplated some of the annoyances to which I have bid farewell.

For one, I no longer hurt or lose my breath just by bending to pull on a pair of socks.

That task would roll my stomach fat atop itself and crush it when the upper and lower sections of my body approached each other, as is necessary to reach a foot with a hand.

For another, I don't bang my bones when passing through standard-size doorways or between obstacles that, to my mind, are easily passable.

I also can zip up a flight of stairs without grabbing a railing and gasping for air. I mean, I never expected to have the endurance of a marathon runner, but simply waddling upward should not cause such a beating. It no longer does.

It is tempting to compare that duty with strapping on a backpack of 70 pounds. That analogy is incorrect, however. It is much easier for a person of proper weight and normal health to "carry" dead weight under stress (uphill) than it is for a person who has 70 pounds of fat dispersed among his bones, muscles and cardiovascular system because the latter is so inordinately more burdening while trying to make the climb.

Skin tags... They've vanished. Medical science is still studying the link between obesity and the small, useless, epidermal slabs but suggests they are more abundant in overweight and older people.

All I know is mine are gone and I have gotten no younger.

The threat of diabetes...? Canceled.

I no longer feel shame when I remove my shirt in public. I did it recently at the beach. No one screamed. No one ran.

I can paddle around on my surfboard without my wetsuit constricting my flabby arms, snapping them to my sides and causing me to get worn out within minutes of entering the water.

Smaller clothes and shrinking hats cost less.

I have more energy to chase or escape the wrath of my kids.

My new attitude allows me to concentrate and focus on ways to prosper and enjoy the rest of my days.

I also have no more fear of suffering a sudden heart attack. I am unable to substantiate actual removal of any danger that existed. I only can say the fright I once had is gone.

Only a person with way too much fat on the body knows what it is like to believe that the heart could give out at any minute without warning—that a complete collapse lurks just beyond the next plate of pasta.

Only genetics and other physical factors can foretell the odds of such a catastrophic event, but I am living my life like there is a tomorrow and it allows me to enjoy my family and everything else so much more.

I have every reason to believe I will be around to see my kids reach adulthood.

If you are reading this before beginning your diet program, I wish you the best of luck in your pursuit of great health.

Please do not rely on luck, though. You will most certainly succeed if you follow the instructions of the program without variation.

You will be amazed at how simple and easy it is to drop the unwanted fat. Stick with the program and you will be thrilled with the new you, guaranteed.

If you have followed along during your diet and have remained within the program parameters, I would like to congratulate you on your success.

The days, months and years ahead will be so much more enjoyable with your new body and improved health.

Regardless of where you may be in your diet program, I invite you to continue gaining knowledge and receiving motivational support at the website, www.FlablesslyFit.com.

There you will find articles on food, nutrition, fitness and other topics of interest to folks like us who want to keep our bodies in shape for the rest of our lives.

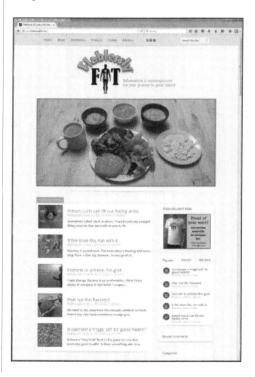

You also can suggest articles, comment and share your stories with other people at various stages in their pursuits of fitness.

Also, if you "like" us on Facebook (www.facebook.com/FlablesslyFit), you occasionally will receive a notification in your Facebook news feed that a new article has been posted to the website.

I look forward to your joining us on the internet and to hearing from you soon.

One last thing!

If you believe this book was helpful to you or you think it might be beneficial to a friend or someone else considering a diet program, please help spread the word and go to your favorite online retailer to provide a review. Your efforts will be most appreciated.

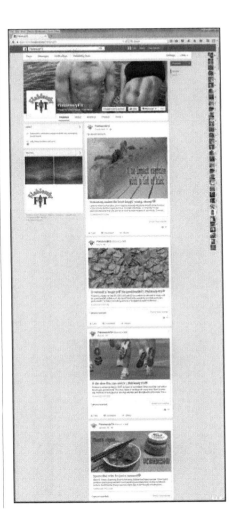

Packaged Foods

This program permits dieters to eat any of its packaged foods in any order desired as long as the prescribed number of meals is not surpassed.

The company shelves are heavily stocked with an array of selections. The meals I describe below are only a sampling of the offerings.

These are items I tried and thought my notes on them would benefit the reader by providing some advance information.

I would suggest you try others, too, in accordance with your estimated preferences.

Macaroni & Cheese

This is quite similar to the standard "mac & cheese" that many parents give to their children on a regular basis. It is not close enough, however, to make an adult eat it regularly, even for purposes of this diet. It is suitable on occasion to diverge from your routine so you feel you have more variety in your selections. That is about it, though.

Scrambled Eggs

If you are a fan of natural eggs in their "scrambled" form, you may consider this to be a perfect replacement. I found no discernable difference between the true item and this program's packaged version. Even the color was appropriate. I added some salt and thought I was eating a routine, pre-diet breakfast. The diet edition has much less cholesterol, however.

Brownie Soft Bake

This was one of my favorites and became a staple in my daily routine. I only cooked it once, however, as it was even better when eaten in its mixed-dough form.

Cappuccino

I used this drink as a replacement for my morning coffee because my creamer failed to meet the program specifications. This offering was so good I was worried I would need to continue purchasing the packets long after I completed the diet. It has a flavor that is difficult to explain. Just give it a try and see if you find it to be incredible.

Oatmeal, Cinnamon Apple

This was acceptable. It certainly was not my favorite, but that is only because of the particulars of the flavor. The texture of this meal does not

match its relatives, the old fashioned variety, however. So, if you have experience with the whole grain stuff, you may wish to forego this instant version.

Oatmeal, Maple Brown Sugar

Since I had no history of eating oatmeal when I began this diet program, I was unable to compare this meal to the "real" thing. The mushy, mashed-potato-type texture of this instant meal was no problem for me and I really enjoyed the flavor. It quickly became a regular item in my daily lineup. Also, co-workers always commented favorably about the aroma wafting through the halls whenever I cooked a batch in the microwave near my office.

Vegetable Chili

This is a serious contender for being a regular part of a dieter's routine. All I can say is try it at least once to see how it fares with your palate.

Peanut Butter Crunch Bar

This is a great snack. It was a regular part of my daily diet until I discovered the

Chocolate Crunch Bar. Even thereafter, I periodically entered the peanut butter version into my program schedule to provide some welcomed variety.

Dutch Chocolate Shake

This drink is better than I expected from a water-based mixture. It is quite rich and flavorful. I didn't drink it on a regular basis, however, since it is supposed to be made with crushed ice. I found that ingredient to be a hassle to produce. So, I either drank it straight or chose something else.

Peanut Butter Soft Serve

This offering is quite enjoyable. Its texture is similar to ice cream or frozen yogurt like you can get from commercial vendors. It suffers, however, from the need to crush and blend ice into the mix to achieve the consistency called for in the instructions. It can be "eaten" in its soupy form, if you have no suitable blender or willingness to take the time to concoct the thing in accordance with the manufacturer's intentions.

Vegetarian Sloppy Joe

I love this meal. There is no way to know the ingredients contain no meat. It is exactly like the Sloppy Joe mix I ate as a kid, minus the bread bun. This became a regular part of my day and remained so for a large portion of my program.

Chocolate Crunch Bar

Oh, my goodness! If you are a chocolate lover like I am, this is an absolute MUST. You may even find yourself eating it more than once a day. I think I would consider it my top choice among the program offerings. Enjoy!

Lemon Meringue Crunch Bar

This is certainly a viable choice for your plan. You will decide according to your taste buds. I was initially excited by the name because I related it to the pie of similar description. The crunch bar misses the full richness of its counterpart, however. Still, I ate the bar every now and then for variety, but I found it easily less "habit-forming" than either the chocolate or peanut butter versions.

Chocolate Pudding

This is every bit as good in flavor as store-bought pudding. You can chill it in your refrigerator or eat it immediately after mixing. Either way, the taste is enjoyable. What keeps it from being a favorite of mine was my inability to get it mixed to a uniform consistency. No matter how much I tried, I always failed to get the lumps out. Good luck on that.

Ziti Marinara

This is a good meal. It probably will fall a bit short of your expectations for pasta, however. There are somewhat few noodles in the package and your mind will be prepared for a full belly afterward, if you have experience with the original, Italian-style edition. It is no complete letdown, however, and I would suggest giving it a try. I enjoyed this meal at regular intervals.

Fruit & Nut Crunch Bar

I suppose this is a good selection, if you normally enjoy this type of snack. I gave it a try and found the flavor to be enjoyable. I am not a fan of the squishy, chewiness of raisins, however, and this contained something that gave that feel when I ate it. So, I steered clear of it after my first endeavor.

Garlic Mashed Potatoes

This meal tastes great, no doubt about it. I enjoyed it thoroughly. The only reason it wasn't a staple in my plan was because I found other items to be more attractive for their ability to make me feel full. I highly recommend this, though, as an addition to a regular meal that normally includes such a thing. For example, I added it to my turkey dish at Thanksgiving. It helped make the meal seem closer to the traditional plate I have enjoyed since I was a child.

Pre-Made "Normal" Meals

(Turkey Meatball Marinara; Chicken Cacciatore; Chicken with Rice and Vegetables)

These are all fine meals. They are intended to be only an occasional stand-in for the program's one daily "normal" meal that a program dieter prepares and eats at home. Each of these packaged offerings is about 300 calories

and tastes great. They are very
convenient and it is possible
to rely too heavily on them.
They are processed food,
however, and should only be
eaten when you have no other
choice. I enjoyed them for
a few days in the beginning
of my program. They helped
greatly before I was able to
make a thorough shopping
trip to purchase all the items I
would need for eating properly
at my dinner table. Once
my shelves were adequately
stocked, I shifted to the
wholesome meals and never
looked back.

89125066R00141

Made in the USA
Lexington, KY
23 May 2018